D1650218

* 7 9 2 5 *

Dementia and Mental Illness in the Old

This book is to be returned on or before
the last date stamped below.

21/4/11

MURPHY, Elaine

THE BRITISH SCHOOL OF OSTEOPATHY
1-4 SUFFOLK ST., LONDON. SW1Y 4HG
TEL. 01 - 930 9254-8

Dementia and Mental Illness in the Old

Elaine Murphy

PAPERMAC

Copyright © Elaine Murphy 1986

All rights reserved. No reproduction, copy or transmission
of this publication may be made without written permission.
No paragraph of this publication may be reproduced, copied or
transmitted save with written permission or in
accordance with the provisions of the Copyright Act 1956
(as amended). Any person who does any unauthorised act
in relation to this publication may be liable to criminal
prosecution and civil claims for damages.

First published 1986 by
PAPERMAC
a division of Macmillan Publishers Limited
4 Little Essex Street London WC2R 3LF
and Basingstoke

Associated companies in Auckland, Delhi, Dublin, Gaborone,
Hamburg, Harare, Hong Kong, Johannesburg, Kuala Lumpur,
Lagos, Manzini, Melbourne, Mexico City, Nairobi, New York,
Singapore and Tokyo

Reprinted 1987 (twice)

British Library Cataloguing in Publication Data
Murphy, Elaine
    Dementia and mental illness in the old.
    1. Presenile dementia——Patients——Home
    care 2. Senile dementia——Patients——
    Home care
    I. Title
    649.8   RC521

    ISBN 0-333-42688-6

Typeset by Columns of Reading
Printed and bound in Great Britain by
Richard Clay Ltd, Bungay, Suffolk

Contents

Preface

Mental problems in old age not only cause much suffering to individuals and their families but are often perplexing and unpredictable. Also, whilst it is difficult for professionals to find their way around the maze of uncoordinated public and voluntary services that are available, this is even more problematic for relatives managing difficult situations on their own. This book was written primarily for relatives, to give them more information about particular mental conditions that affect elderly people and the likely course of events, and also to give some guidance about where to get help, what practical assistance is available and how to drum up support from local services.

There is also of course a vast army of professional helpers providing care to elderly people living in their own homes in the community, and another large group of workers caring for old people living in residential homes and long-stay hospitals. Everyone who comes into contact regularly with elderly people during the course of their work is bound to have to cope with old people who have dementia, confusion or depression. I hope this book will be useful therefore not only to relatives but also to the invaluable battalions of home helps, meals-on-wheels organisers, social welfare officers, care assistants, nursing auxiliaries, residential social work staff and housing advisers for the elderly. Trained staff such as social workers and district nurses may perhaps also find this book useful 'refresher' reading. There is also now a growing band of volunteers who run clubs, day centres and a wide range of other activities for old people. They are eager to provide the best possible service and want to know more about this particularly challenging group.

One of my colleagues suggested that the title of this book should be 'Keeping Mum'. Women survive longer than men as a general rule, so there are far more women than men suffering from mental problems in old age. Throughout this book therefore I have usually referred to the sufferer as 'she', but the reader must remember that men are also likely to suffer from the same problems and will need exactly the same kind of help. For similar reasons of convenience I have referred to all doctors as 'he' and to all social workers and nurses as 'she'. As a female doctor who works with many male nurses and social workers I am aware that these stereotypes are long out of date, but the English language insists that we choose.

I should like to add a final note of thanks to Eileen Chandler, who typed the manuscript.

Elaine Murphy
London, February 1986

1

Mental Illness in Old Age: an Introduction

Winston Churchill was seventy-seven years old when he retired as Prime Minister in 1955, a vastly changed man from the person who had led Britain through the Second World War. He was suffering from the early stages of dementia. Lord Moran, his personal physician, carefully documented the course of the symptoms, giving us an excellent account of the progress of Churchill's physical and mental health. The very earliest problems were first noticed in the later years of the Second World War. At times Churchill had difficulty concentrating on official papers, and his mind occasionally wandered off the topic at important meetings. Field Marshal Alanbrooke remarked in March 1944 that Churchill seemed scarcely able to concentrate for longer than a few minutes. Several other observers noted that he appeared over-tired and unlike his old self. He was sometimes quarrelsome and irritable, and consequently his relationships with some of his key allies deteriorated. He argued with Roosevelt and never re-established a good relationship with him.

These vague early signs mean little on their own. Churchill was after all carrying a great burden of responsibility and was under great stress all the time. However, four years after the war was over, one evening in August 1949, Churchill suffered a mild stroke. He had spent the evening playing cards in Monte Carlo and returning home late found that his right hand and arm felt weak and heavy. He became shaky on his feet and had difficulty walking. He recovered very quickly from this mild stroke, and the whole thing was carefully hushed up so as not to reach the public ear. Within the next two years there were two further mild episodes during which his speech was affected for a few hours, but again he made a quick recovery.

By the time he returned triumphantly to No. 10 Downing Street in 1951, however, Churchill was already suffering from a decline in his mental functions. This man who had previously been able to work all hours with intense concentration could at times not follow the drift of conversations or grasp the meaning of official documents. His private secretary condensed down long documents to a single paragraph. Churchill appeared to lose his self-confidence and ability to make major decisions. His memory for what was happening in the world around him was poor. Yet he steadfastly denied that anything was wrong with him and resisted all suggestions that he rest or step down from the job. He had a further stroke in June 1953. This time it couldn't be hidden from the public because it occurred during a state banquet. Once again he made a good physical recovery. For a while he preserved his public façade and rehearsed his speeches well. Outside the close circle of the Cabinet, his colleagues and his family, few would have guessed that anything was seriously amiss. However, within a year he began to make serious errors when speaking in public and became confused over names and places. Then in 1955 he was persuaded to step down in favour of his deputy, Anthony Eden, to the great relief of those around him. He lived for another ten years, his mental state declining further until he became immobile and seriously forgetful, and needed a good deal of physical nursing care.

Winston Churchill suffered from one of the commonest conditions of old age: dementia caused by disease of the arteries in the brain. Dementia and other mental illnesses in old age can happen to anyone and are extremely common in the general population. There are now more than 1½ million people in Britain suffering from one of the major mental disorders of old age. This book is for their relatives and friends and for those who work with elderly people – indeed, for anyone who wants to know more about the problems of mental disorder in old age. The causes, symptoms and effects of the disorders will be described and then some of the practical ways in which sufferers and their families can be helped. Let us first set the problem in the context of the elderly population as a whole.

Are old people living longer these days?

It has been estimated that two out of every three elderly people who have ever lived on this earth are alive today. This startling idea is suggested by looking at the age structure of the population of developed Western European countries over the past eighty years. At the beginning of the century, in 1901, there were 200,000 women over the age of seventy-five years in the United Kingdom. By the year 2001 the number will be five times as large, something over a million. The population of old people has grown faster than the population of young people, so we now have a society in which there is a rising percentage of old people and a falling percentage of young and middle-aged people. Elderly people over sixty-five years now make up 15 per cent of the population, whereas at the turn of the century the figure was only 4 per cent, so there are many more elderly people around than ever before.

Elderly people are also living longer. More than at any other time in history, a person has a good chance of surviving into their eighties, nineties and beyond. There are now at least 3,000 centenarians in Britain. The main change in the age structure of the population came about as a result of improvements in sanitation, nutrition and general living conditions towards the end of the nineteenth century. Improved living standards caused a dramatic fall in the number of babies who died at birth or in early childhood. Most members of the large Victorian and Edwardian families now began to survive the hazards of childhood and live to a ripe old age.

A further change then occurred. As people's living standards improved they produced fewer children. They planned their families more carefully, surer than previous generations that most of their children would survive to adulthood. This happened all over Western Europe and the developed world. The number of births began to fall at the end of the last century, and this overall pattern has continued through our own century. Two children are now considered a fair size for a complete family, whereas in the Middle Ages and up until the late nineteenth century it was thought desirable to have as many children as possible to ensure that at least one or two would survive. Thus a fall in the birth rate, most children surviving to adulthood and an increased life expectancy have all led to a population in which there is a large proportion of elderly people.

Parts of Western Europe, notably Scandinavia and the United Kingdom, have the highest proportions of elderly anywhere in the world. The United States and Canada, Japan and the rest of Europe are catching up fast but still do not have quite as ageing a population as ours is. In this respect, at least, Britain is a world leader.

Extent of the problem of mental illness in old age

The majority of elderly people remain mentally well until the end of their days. Four out of five pensioners over the age of eighty-five have no problems with their memories and can concentrate with as much vigour and energy as they ever could. This means that you and I have a very good chance of remaining alert and 'in our right minds' even in great old age. There are dozens of very old people in their eighties and nineties still pursuing an active, independent life. Take the example of another twentieth-century Prime Minister, Harold Macmillan. In 1984 he entered the House of Lords as the Earl of Stockton at the age of ninety. His maiden speech to the Lords was delivered with a clarity and enthusiasm that many novice MPs in their thirties would have envied. He spoke to the point, from memory, for ninety minutes, entirely without notes. He is not exceptional. There are far more elderly people with all their faculties intact than there are suffering from mental decline or 'senility'.

We all have preconceived ideas about groups of people who we do not come into contact with very much – about different racial or national groups, for example. As soon as we get to know individuals from another culture we perceive how wrong our stereotyped opinions were. Our preconceived notions about elderly people are often similarly wrong. Younger people often fear that old age will be a slow decline into mental and physical inactivity, a period of loneliness, poverty and misery. Shakespeare said it all when he described the 'seven ages of man' in *As You Like It*:

> . . . Last scene of all,
> That ends this strange eventful history,
> Is second childishness, and mere oblivion,
> Sans teeth, sans eyes, sans taste, sans everything.

Curiously, old people often share this pessimistic view of what life is like for other old people but feel they are just the lucky ones who have avoided the worst. By and large however this view of old age is inaccurate for the vast majority of elderly people.

One of the problems about a book like this one is that it concentrates on the very real and serious mental health problems that affect the minority. There is a danger that the reader will get the idea that mental decline is the inevitable consequence of ageing. Younger people who work with the elderly in hospitals, old people's homes and day centres can get a biased view of what old age is like for most people. They never see the independent, fit, healthy ones taking care of themselves and living an active, happy, fulfilling old age. So if you have a relative or friend causing concern or you work with elderly people with mental health problems, remember they are the exceptions.

Exceptional though they may be in terms of proportions,

the *numbers* of elderly people with mental illness do pose very serious problems for their families, for neighbours and for the health and social services provided by the state. Mental illness is now the primary reason for someone going to live in an old people's home, nursing home or long-stay hospital.

In the United Kingdom, out of 8 million elderly people over the age of sixty-five, approximately one in ten, or 800,000, have some form of dementia, serious confusion as a result of physical illness or serious psychiatric illness requiring hospital treatment. To this figure must be added another 800,000 who are mentally alert but whose lives are made a misery by serious depression that would benefit from treatment. These figures are rising rapidly because of the growth of the population over eighty-five years old, since it is these 'very, very old' who are most at risk of developing serious mental disorder.

Where are all the elderly people?

Nearly a third of elderly people now live alone in their own homes, and most of those who live alone are women. (Because men tend to die younger than women, there is a preponderance of elderly widowed women left on their own. Only 17 per cent of elderly men live alone because most still live with their wives, whereas nearly a half of elderly women live alone.) Overall, about one-third of the elderly live with their husband or wife, one-third (mostly women) live alone, a little less than a third live with family or friends, and only 6 per cent live in hospitals, homes or in residential care.

The small proportion of elderly people in residential care sometimes surprises people. The UK has a lower proportion of old people living in institutions than anywhere else in Europe. This is partly because of government policy, which has restricted the growth of old people's homes and long-term hospital beds; but it also largely reflects the wishes of old people themselves, who want to continue to live in ordinary accommodation like the rest of us for as long as possible.

There has been a lot of discussion about the government's policy of 'care in the community'. This policy places emphasis upon helping elderly people at home and is designed to prevent unnecessary permanent admission to homes and hospitals. There are some who complain that this is the wrong policy and that we ought to press for the growth of hospital and institutional care. But in the UK we have never had a policy of encouraging elderly people to enter long-term care. We have always had 'care in the community' whether we like it or not. The difference now is that for the last fifteen years the government has realised that sufficient help and support ought to be provided for elderly people and their families if they are going to cope satisfactorily in their own homes.

The extent of the need was shown clearly by the General Household Survey of 1980, which found that 12 out of every 100 elderly people were unable to get out of the house and walk down the road alone, and 7 of these 12 could not get out of the house even with help from someone else; 2 out of these 7 totally housebound old people were permanently bed-ridden.

Think about what these figures mean across the country. Nearly a million old people are now dependent on other people to do their shopping, collect their pensions and do major jobs around the house. The degree of disability increases dramatically over the age of eighty-five. A half of all old people over eighty-five are unable to go out of doors and walk up the road unaided or to get upstairs and downstairs alone. Considerably more than one-third of these very old people are unable to bath, shower or wash all over by themselves. Much of this dependence on others is of course caused through physical handicap as a result of physical illness, but mental disorder is an important cause of loss of independence.

Who looks after old people?

Most old people look after themselves without much help from anyone else. But what of those who do need help: who looks after them? It is often said that old age is nowadays particularly characterised by loneliness and isolation from others and that old people are now more neglected by their relatives when they grow frail – 'Old people aren't looked after by their families like they used to be.' I often hear this said by people who believe there was some golden age, before the world wars, before married women worked outside the home, when old people were nurtured in the bosom of their family. We can conjure up an idyllic scene of rosy-cheeked, cheery old folk sitting happily by the hearth surrounded by their stalwart families. All the evidence suggests that life in Britain was never like this.

First, there were never very many old people around until the twentieth century. The few people who did survive into old age certainly did become dependent on their families when they were unable to continue work unless they belonged to the richer classes. But old people from the poorer labouring classes have not always been welcome in the homes of their children and of course they did not all have children surviving who could take care of them. The parish records of 'outdoor relief', public charity money from the parish purse, are eloquent evidence that the old and poor never lived in a golden age.

In the nineteenth century old people who were not supported by their families and were not managing on 'outdoor relief' either entered an almshouse (sheltered flats are our modern equivalent) where folk cared largely for themselves, or were forced to enter the parish workhouse or asylum. Residents of the Poor Law workhouses were the poor, the chronically sick, the handicapped or disabled, the mentally ill and anyone of any age who could not support themselves. As the nineteenth century wore on, the workhouses came to be largely occupied by old people because of the ever-increasing numbers with no one to care for them. These institutions were designed to discourage people from wanting to enter them, on the pious principle that the poor would have no incentive to provide for themselves if comfortable conditions were provided by charity. One Assistant Commissioner of the Poor Law wrote: 'Our object is to establish therein a discipline so severe and repulsive as to make them a terror to the poor and prevent them from entering.' A similar argument is used nowadays to keep the level of unemployment benefit down to the minimum possible.

But public concern about the conditions of the poor was stimulated by the work of the great reformers at the end of the last century. The Royal Commission on the Poor Laws Minority Report (1909) made the following points:

> There ought to be some practical method by which a helpless old person may escape from or protect herself against the tyranny and repeated petty cruelties to which the aged are sometimes subjected, even by their own children. There should be for all cases, available in every district, asylums or retreats under a more accurate and less degrading title than that of workhouse and under less stringent and kinder disciplines.

So much for the golden age when all families cared for their own old people.

How isolated are elderly people from their families?

What about now? The overwhelming majority of elderly people in Britain have regular contact with relatives, friends and neighbours. One-third see a relative or friend every day, another third see a close friend or relative two or three times a week and another quarter see someone close once a week. Of those who live alone, a third have a close relative living near by whom they see frequently. Three per cent of old people have no contact with relatives and friends at all, and 10 per cent do not have any contact with their neighbours; so there is a minority who have to rely for any help they need on public and voluntary services. However, for the large majority of elderly people needing help, this help is provided by *relatives*. The reality of 'community care' is that it is largely family care. This means in practice female care provided by wives, daughters and daughters-in-law.

There are no reliable statistics about the numbers of such 'carers' in Britain, but it has been estimated that there are now about 1¼ million, the majority of whom are women looking after an elderly dependent relative. *There are now more women caring for old people than there are women caring for babies.* The average age of the main carer is now more than sixty, and carers often need a substantial amount of help because they themselves may be in poor health. Half of all married women can expect at some time or another to give practical help to an elderly or infirm person. So if you are a carer, take some comfort from the fact that you have plenty of company.

Well over three-quarters of the main supporters of elderly confused people are women, but we must not forget the other quarter who are men, who often have to learn domestic and nursing skills late in life in order to cope. But men seem to get more help when they have a dependent person to care for than do women. An elderly man looking after a confused wife is more likely to be allocated a home help, for example, than an elderly woman looking after a confused husband. The reasons are not hard to fathom. Society expects women to be nurses and carers; after all, this is what bringing up small children is about. There is a belief that for women nurturing skills come naturally. Men on the other hand are not supposed to take on this role as a matter of course, particularly in late life. Furthermore, when they do, they receive society's approval and praise more readily than women. Men who give up paid work to care for an elderly parent are entitled to an invalid care allowance to compensate them for loss of earnings. Married women who do the same are not entitled to claim a penny. This is one area of women's rights that needs a serious rethink if 'community care' is to work satisfactorily. Fortunately, such a rethink seems now to be happening.

What kinds of mental disorder affect old people – is it just senility?

There are four groups of mental conditions described in this book, two of which are caused by physical illness in the brain (the dementias and acute confusional states) and two that occur in mentally alert old people (depressions and paranoid illnesses). When people talk of someone 'going senile' or 'confused' they are usually referring to a progressive decline of mental faculties in old age for which the medical term is *dementia*. Dementia can occur at any age and is occasionally found in people in their fifties and sixties, although the main sufferers are elderly people over the age of seventy-five.

Acute confusional state is the term used to describe the sudden confusion that results from acute physical illness elsewhere in the body, or as an adverse reaction to medication, or due to some other sudden upset to the body's delicate metabolic balance. People usually recover completely from an acute confusional state, whereas someone suffering from dementia does not recover.

Depression can occur at any age and is common in old age. It is a more frequent problem than dementia. Paranoid illnesses, on the other hand, are rare but when they do crop up they tend to cause a great deal of difficulty for the sufferer, for her neighbours and for relatives.

Dementia has been given far more space in this book than any of the other conditions. This is because an elderly person with dementia needs an enormous amount of help from relatives, neighbours and statutory services, and help is often difficult to come by. Whether the reader is a husband caring for a wife with dementia, a daughter-in-law struggling with an elderly man after a stroke, or a home help who provides the main day-to-day practical care for a frail confused person at home, I hope you will find here some useful information on how to manage the problems better.

2

Dementia

What is dementia?

'Dementia' is a frightening word. It conjures up pictures of wild-eyed people running amok, violent and deranged. Nothing could be further from the truth. Whilst it is true that dementia means 'loss of mind', in medical terminology it denotes a group of progressive diseases of the brain that slowly affect all the functions of the mind and lead to a deterioration in a person's ability to concentrate, remember and reason. Dementia can affect every area of human thinking, feeling and behaviour. The disease starts silently and very slowly so that it may have been progressing insidiously for two or three years before anyone notices anything seriously amiss. When people refer to an old person as being 'senile' they are usually referring to someone with dementia. Senile just means 'old', however; and since the majority of old people never have any serious mental problems at all, it is not accurate or fair on all the normal old people to lump the two concepts together. Dementia is the specific medical term that refers to a defined group of mental conditions, which can affect people of any age.

It is normal to experience a gradual slowing down of one's mental processes over the course of a lifetime. It is said that mathematicians generally produce their best work when they are relatively young. Flying supersonic jet aircraft calls for a young mind and quick reflexes. Dementia is not normal ageing, however. It is an ageing process that starts gradually to 'knock out' areas of the brain so that they function less well. It can happen in younger people but most commonly occurs in the elderly.

Dementia is not just 'getting old'

The majority of old people remain mentally alert throughout their lives. As we age we of course tend to work things out more slowly, take longer to learn new addresses and phone numbers, and may even from time to time forget the names of relatives or friends. This can be irritating, particularly for the person to whom it is happening, but normal old people don't become seriously forgetful or develop any of the other changes that go with dementia. But if a friend or relative becomes *seriously* forgetful or *seriously* confused, don't let anyone tell you that it is nothing to worry about, 'just old age', because it is not 'just old age'. Dementia is a real illness.

How does dementia show itself?

It can be months or years before the penny drops for relatives. They may have noticed that the elderly person is not so interested as before in things around them, not so concerned about the grandchildren, or she may have given up hobbies. The elderly person may become very much slower to 'catch on' to information and pick up on new ideas. You have to repeat things on the phone. She may frequently forget what you said to her last week. The house is not quite so spick and span as it once was, and clothing does not get changed as often as previously. It all starts so gradually that it is easy to shrug it off, to attribute it to a sort of slowing down. But soon the serious problems emerge.

The symptoms of dementia vary widely from one person to another. The way a person is affected depends on the site and progress of the illness in the brain but also on how the individual personality reacts to and copes with increasing mental impairment. In fact some of the most difficult problems for caring relatives are caused by the person's misjudged attempts to cope with a perplexing experience.

Not all the symptoms to be described in the coming chapters will apply to everyone. Dementia does not necessarily progress rapidly in all cases, and many elderly people in the early stages of dementia appear to remain the same for many years without any further deterioration. So those people reading this book with a relative or friend in mind should not jump to the conclusion that all these problems are inevitable. This is a guide to inform you of all that *can* happen in dementia, and few patients will give rise to all the problems described.

Forgetfulness

Forgetfulness is the direct cause of many of the patient's problems in managing daily life without help. Memory of the recent past – that is, the last few hours, days or weeks – is affected most seriously; but in the early stages of the disease the elderly person often preserves detailed memories of her past life right back to childhood. The consequence of this is that while the person cannot remember where she was yesterday or what she ate for tea two hours ago, she may be able to give an accurate account of her first day at work decades ago. Names of close relatives may also be forgotten, or mixed up. Kettles and saucepans may be left to boil dry, gas taps left turned on without being lit, front doors left unlocked all night – all because of forgetfulness. The person will perhaps forget having put the kettle on to boil or go out shopping and be unable to remember the way back home. As the illness progresses she may be able to remember very little at all beyond a few seconds at a time and may be unable to learn new things. She may, for example, be unable to use the new 'automatic switch off' electric kettle that has been thoughtfully bought to avoid the risk of burning out another one on top of the stove. Memory for the events of the past gradually becomes patchy and confused; names of brothers and sisters and even the name of a husband or wife and children will be forgotten.

Grasp

The person finds it difficult to understand what is happening around her. Grasping what day it is, where she is or who a new visitor is becomes near impossible. This leads to repetitive questions about the time, the day, the date and so on, which may have been answered two minutes earlier or twenty times already that day. She may lose her normal sense of time and wander out at night thinking it is time to do the shopping. She may misinterpret what she sees or hears, for example thinking the person on the television is really in the room.

Personality

Many sufferers of dementia remain more or less their old selves. However, they are inclined to get more easily upset, can get distressed very rapidly and may seem to be less warm and close to the family than before. Sadly, some patients change and become quite different characters, acting in a verbally aggressive and punitive way towards their relatives and becoming suspicious and accusatory. In the worse cases the original personality becomes eroded so much that it is difficult to remember that this is still the same person. Some become permanently perplexed and anxious, constantly seeking reassurance. Others become very changeable, laughing one minute and tearful the next.

Communication

Speech problems are very common in dementia; finding the right word and keeping track of an idea to the end of a sentence become difficult. Sufferers may constantly repeat themselves. Eventually it becomes difficult for them to make sentences at all, and speech is confined to a few words, phrases or questions. If speech deteriorates early, it can be very frustrating for the patient to get others to understand. The patient with dementia also has difficulty in understanding what other people are saying to her.

Behaviour

Dementia leads to wandering and to neglect of personal hygiene, and causes a failure to perform routine household chores. Sufferers may abandon the conventions of polite society, for example by undressing or urinating in public, or by swearing, masturbating openly or indulging in some other form of embarrassing behaviour. The inability to care for oneself leads eventually to dependence on others for dressing, feeding, bathing and using the toilet.

Movement and balance

In the early stages dementia causes no problems in walking, balancing or moving, but as the illness progresses patients tend to shuffle with small steps or walk lopsidedly. They suffer frequent falls and trip over obstacles easily. In the later stages some patients become immobile and physically weak, but this is by no means the general rule.

Chapter 3 describes some of these problems in more detail and offers advice on how to deal with them.

Main causes of dementia?

There are two main types of dementia.

Alzheimer's disease

About half of all people who have dementia have *Alzheimer's disease* (pronounced 'Alts-himer', to rhyme with 'I'm a . . .'). Alzheimer was a German doctor working at the turn of this century who first described the brain changes that are characteristic of the disease. These brain changes can be clearly seen under the microscope. The outer layers of the brain become particularly affected by a wide range of biochemical abnormalities. We know a great deal now about these abnormalities and know that they affect the way nerve cells pass on their messages to other cells. Those parts of the brain concerned with memory and learning are particularly badly affected, as one might expect.

In the last twenty years biochemists and pathologists have greatly advanced our knowledge of the underlying brain changes that occur in Alzheimer's disease. Some very exciting research work is now being done that may give hope of prevention or treatment for the future. Unfortunately the human brain is so staggeringly complex that the benefits of this research are unlikely to be available for many years. All kinds of hypotheses have been suggested as to what causes Alzheimer's disease: something in the diet, a virus or some kind of infection acting over a long period of time. Environmental pollution has also been studied. Sadly, we haven't a clue at this stage as to why some people get dementia and others don't. Perhaps in another ten or fifteen years we will know much more.

Multi-infarct dementia

The other common cause of dementia is usually called *multi-infarct dementia*, which means that the brain has developed multiple small areas of dead tissue. Another term for the same condition is 'cerebrovascular dementia' or 'arteriosclerotic dementia'. All these names are derived from Latin medical words describing the death of small areas of the brain due to small 'strokes' in the brain as a result of blockages forming in small brain arteries.

Multi-infarct dementia is relatively rare, and only one in seven or so of dementia sufferers has this kind of problem. We know that it is commoner in people with a long history of high blood pressure, in those who have had other major strokes affecting their limbs and in people who have had other circulatory problems such as coronary artery disease. People are often surprised to hear that you can have 'strokes' without losing the use of an arm or leg or passing out unconscious, but the effect of a stroke will depend on what part of the brain is affected and how widespread is the damage. Patients often make marvellous recoveries after strokes, and in the early stages of multi-infarct dementia there may be considerable improvement after each small stroke set-back. This is very confusing for those caring for the sufferer as the illness appears irritatingly unpredictable.

Apart from Alzheimer's disease and multi-infarct dementia, there are a number of rare causes of dementia that account for less than 10 per cent of all cases. Some of them are important because they may be treatable. As a general rule, the younger the person afflicted, the more likely it is that the illness will turn out to have an unusual cause.

It is not always straightforward to tell one form of dementia from another, especially when someone has been suffering from the condition for a few years. But medical researchers can tell from looking at the brain after death which illness the patient was suffering. At present the distinction between these two main illnesses is not really helpful in treatment, but it is helpful in research, and research will eventually lead to our overcoming this group of diseases.

What does *not* cause dementia?

Why did this happen to him or her? It is human nature to seek reasons for the catastrophes that happen to us, and relatives often ponder about the cause of the problem. There are a number of mistaken ideas around, which are worth mentioning here.

Dementia is not caused by a bang on the head or a fall

A very severe head injury in a car crash can cause permanent brain damage, and the victim may well have many of the same problems as an elderly person with dementia; but there is no evidence that the everyday dementias of the elderly are caused through injuries. Some professional boxers, particularly those who fought in the days when there were few controls over the number of fights that one person could take part in, are also liable to have brain damage caused by multiple blows to the head, but the symptoms are different.

Dementia is not due to laziness or to not using the brain

It is a common fallacy that if you keep your brain active it won't let you down in old age. Dementia affects office workers, dustmen, professors, authors and housewives alike. Thinkers and dunces, dreamers and doers are just as much at risk. A patient's wife once remarked: 'He never seemed to use his brain after he retired – never got himself interested in a hobby or took an interest in anything.' But this probably reflects the silent part of the illness just beginning rather than a triggering cause.

Dementia is not caused through a sudden change

Bereavement, sudden physical illness, moving house and retirement are major events in our lives to which we have to learn to adapt. Dementia is often revealed by an event that exposes the problem. If a husband who has been caring for his demented wife suddenly dies, the extent of her need for care and inability to cope by herself may become quickly obvious to relatives and neighbours. Careful enquiry usually reveals that the stressful event has highlighted the problem but that the dementia was progressing before the event.

Dementia is not catching

Medical textbooks are full of 'curiosities', very rare diseases that most doctors will never ever come across. There was, for example, a famous type of dementia found only in New

Guinea, called *kuru*, caused by an infection caught by taking part in the ritual cannibalism of another infected person. Kuru is fortunately now extinct, but the existence of this extraordinary disease led to a search for infective causes of other dementias. Sure enough there is evidence that one of the extremely rare progressive dementias that affect younger people may be due to a virus which acts very slowly, taking several years to cause the brain damage. Oddly, even this kind of dementia (which has an even more difficult-to-pronounce German name *Creutzfeldt-Jakob disease*) is not very 'catching' and is not easily passed on by contact with another person. The idea that a virus or other infection may cause Alzheimer's disease continues to interest researchers. However, there is not at present any evidence that dementia is due to an infection, and it is certain that you cannot catch dementia by living in the same house as, or being near, the sufferer.

Syphilis, a sexually transmitted disease, if not properly treated, can cause a type of dementia after twenty to thirty years. This used to be relatively common in the earlier years of this century but is now thankfully rare. However, it is still common practice for doctors to do a simple routine screening blood test for syphilis on most patients, because this kind of dementia can be improved with penicillin, and it would be foolish to omit such a simple test even if the chances of finding such a case are one in a million.

Dementia is not inherited

The chances of a son or daughter of an affected person developing dementia are no higher in general than for the rest of the population. If an elderly relative of yours develops senile dementia, there is no need to worry about yourself or your children. There are a few families that have a history of dementia starting early in middle age, but even in these families the risk to children is small. Ordinary senile dementia and multi-infarct dementia are not inherited.

How long will it go on for?

Dementia does not get better and almost always gets worse. The brain's function is gradually destroyed. There is no effective treatment that will slow down or halt the progress of the illness, and most patients eventually die directly or indirectly from the illness. In this sense dementia is a 'terminal' illness. But it is extremely difficult to predict how fast the illness will progress or how long the patient will live. It used to be said that by the time someone was so severely disabled that they needed care in a hospital, the majority of patients would have less than two years to live. But this was an *average* length of time and there was enormous variability between one person and another. Somewhat paradoxically, the younger the person at the onset of the condition, the more rapid the decline. An 85-year-old may therefore live a lot longer and deteriorate more slowly than a 65-year-old with the same type of illness. However, it is usual for the illness to last between two and ten years.

Seeking medical advice

What is the point of going to the doctor about the problem if there is no cure for dementia? There are several very good reasons. Most important, there are many conditions that superficially have the same symptoms as dementia but are really separate illnesses that can be treated. It is difficult to distinguish some kinds of severe depression from dementia. Confusion caused by physical illness may also outwardly resemble dementia. (Even young people can become confused when they have a physical illness.)

Second, as already mentioned, there are rare causes of dementia that are treatable. A good physical examination and some blood tests will pick up most of these rare causes. Infections, nutritional deficiencies, thyroid gland disorders and brain tumours can all be treated. *Dementia starting before the age of seventy is very uncommon and should always be medically investigated.*

Third, someone with dementia living alone may have been eating a very poor diet for many months or years. Meals of bread and jam or sweet biscuits are much easier to prepare and eat than a proper cooked meal, but far less nourishing. A poor diet can cause anaemia and vitamin deficiencies, which may make the dementia seem worse than it really is. It is a fairly simple matter to detect these deficiencies and treat them with supplements to the diet.

Fourth, a family doctor can refer the patient to a hospital specialist who has special expertise in these problems and may well have a team of professionals who can give advice and support to the person who gives the day-to-day care. Chapter 5 gives more details about the kind of help that the specialist services can offer.

Fifth, the person who is looking after an elderly person with dementia is under a great deal of strain. 'Going it alone' without professional help and support is a worrying, lonely business. Your doctor should be able to provide that support.

3

Dementia:
Some Problems and
Suggestions on How to
Deal with Them

It is surprising how often the same problems crop up when dealing with people with dementia. In spite of the fact that this book stresses the individual and his or her unique reaction to the predicament of failing mental powers, similar symptoms and difficulties are found in many patients. This is not to say that one person gets all of the problems at once; one or two are more than enough to cope with. Also, many patients never develop the more troublesome symptoms. None the less, it is as well to be forewarned about the worst.

General points on tactics

Developing the right approach to managing your relative's problems is partly a matter of trial and error, learning from past experience what works for you and your relative and what does not. There are few hard and fast rules; after all, you know your relative best. The following are ideas gleaned from talking to people who have coped successfully with the problems.

Getting the priorities right

Most of us have a fixed routine in life and live by a set of social conventions. We get up, wash, dress, eat certain foods for breakfast and go off to work, politely standing in the bus queue, behaving in a generally orderly manner until the end of the day. Some social conventions are concerned with the practical matters of keeping healthy and pleasant to be near (washing, bathing, wearing clean clothes and so on). Other conventions are habits that society imposes on us for quite different reasons – to oil the wheels of personal relationships in the home and at work. For example, the times we get up and go to bed, the times we eat meals, eating with a knife and fork, getting undressed for bed – all these are relatively unimportant routines that we take for granted. You may be surprised to learn that the great literary figure of the eighteenth century, Dr Sam Johnson, frequently got up at four or five in the morning and was in bed by six in the evening. This was his winter schedule, one that most of his contemporaries followed because of the difficulties of working by candle-light.

When you are working with a dementia sufferer you should try to be equally *flexible*, to decide what is important. Learn to take events in a relaxed way, to go with the tide. Does it really matter if something is done another way? If the person will not sit down to eat a meal, try to let her eat while she is walking around. If she won't get in the bath one day, don't worry; try an all-over wash instead. Do not make an issue out of unimportant things.

Accept that your relative *will* change. Last week she may have been able to dress herself with help; this week you may find that her cardigan has been put on inside out and back to front. She may get it right tomorrow but possibly she will not, so don't expect too much. Remember that she may need more help as time goes by.

Whereas the caring person must be flexible, reacting to sudden changes and reverses in the patient's mood with calm, it helps if you can avoid sudden changes of routine in the daily timetable of the patient – getting up, meals, outings, bedtimes and so on. A predictable routine can be reassuring because it is easier to remember.

Try also not to be too protective. Let the person have a go at helping herself to do things and let her continue to practise old skills even if this is slow and difficult. It is tempting to dress someone rather than merely guide and assist. Watching someone struggling with buttons and laces can be very frustrating, particularly if you are feeling rushed and impatient. In the long run, however, the person will become more heavily dependent on you for everything much more quickly if you don't allow her to practise daily skills. There is a knack in knowing when to rescue someone from total failure by offering help, however. At that point the best approach is, 'Shall we try to do this together?' rather than, 'You'd better let me do that if you can't.'

Getting the message across and understanding needs

As mental faculties decline, so does the ability of the sufferer to understand what is said to her. It becomes increasingly difficult too for the patient to make her own wishes understood. Communication is made even more difficult if hearing and sight are impaired. Not so long ago I watched a nurse wheeling a tea-trolley past the end of a bed in a geriatric ward. She stopped at the foot of the bed and asked the elderly woman in the bed, 'Cup of tea?' at a distance of eight feet. The deaf and partially sighted patient answered, 'I've had my medicines already, thank you.' The trolley was whisked away to the next bed, and the nurse turned to me, commenting, 'See, she's very confused!' It turned out that all the patient needed was a good hearing-aid.

It is not always so easy to remedy communication difficulties with a person who has dementia. We often seem to have conversations at cross purposes that go nowhere, leaving both parties feeling frustrated and irritated. How then can you improve your communicating skills?

Hearing

Can she hear you? If not, try speaking loudly and clearly, but not shouting, first in one ear, then the other. Usually one ear is much better than the other. Sit where the person can see your mouth moving. If you haven't been understood first time, repeat the same words, rather than try to introduce new words. Introduce only one idea at a time and give the person time for it to sink in. For example, don't say, 'Now put on your socks and shoes,' but rather, 'Put this sock on this foot now.' If there is just one idea to hear, there is only one idea to grasp and act on.

Hearing-aids

Hearing-aids can help. It is worth having an opinion from a specialist in this field even for someone who is confused. Remember that the elderly person herself will not necessarily be able to manage the aid very well. A relative will need to understand how it works, how to clean it and how to fit it in the ear. A word of caution, though: hearing-aids are difficult to get used to. With normal hearing, our brains filter out a lot of loud background noises – for instance, traffic – as well as the ordinary hurly-burly noises of everyday life. This allows us to focus on conversation, on the television or radio, or on whatever we want to hear. With a hearing-aid all these background sounds are magnified, and the hearing-aid user has to learn consciously to filter out the excess background noise. This is a task that grows more difficult as we age and may be nearly impossible for a person with dementia. But the other side of the coin is that just as deafness can be misinterpreted as lack of understanding, so failure of the brain to grasp the meaning of words may easily be misinterpreted as deafness; deafness hinders communication and understanding in only a minority of cases in dementia.

Hearing-aids are available through the National Health Service or from a private supplier. Before going too far along this road it is best to ask your doctor to check the ears for wax, since this is a common problem easily solved. If there is a real problem that a hearing-aid might solve, there are some very good aids available. But do not spend a lot of money on one before you are convinced that your relative will be willing to wear it and will really benefit. Private hearing-aid consultants make their money from the sale of hearing-aids, and are unlikely to advise you against buying one. Private suppliers are listed in the Yellow Pages of the telephone directory.

For a deaf person living alone you can also consider having specially loud bells fitted to the phone and doorbell, or flashing light bulbs rigged up as a substitute. These are worth considering only if the deaf person can understand the meaning of the flashing light or the ringing bell.

Dementia can sometimes play tricks. A sufferer whose hearing is perfectly normal may be unable to understand spoken words but occasionally retains the ability to understand written words. It is worth trying writing out a message to see if it is understood better, even if the person is not deaf.

Sight

We all become increasingly 'long-sighted' as we age and have more difficulty reading small print. The elderly are also likely to develop two other common causes of poor sight: *cataract*, a clouding of the lens of the eye, and *glaucoma*, increased pressure of the fluid inside the eyeball. Both these problems can be treated, cataract by the right spectacles or by operation, glaucoma by tablets and eye-drops. It is important to treat these conditions early to prevent blindness. Poor sight together with failing understanding is a combination that frequently leads to misinterpretations and distortions of the world around. For example, patterns on the wallpaper appear to be human faces, shadows in the window seem to be ghost-like figures. These problems and 'seeing things' are discussed later in this chapter (page 48).

A word of warning about cataract operations: these are quick, easy operations that are usually a great success. However, a person with memory problems or confusion is likely to be worse immediately after the operation, and you should discuss the patient's dementia problems with the doctor in the out-patient clinic before the operation. A cataract removal is not a sudden miracle cure. On the contrary, it can take weeks for the eyes to adapt to using a new set of spectacles, and a mentally impaired person will take even longer than usual.

Remember also that when the patient says, 'I can't see', it may also mean, 'I can't take it in.' The right spectacles will not necessarily allow her to take up reading or watching TV again.

Getting in touch

Conversations are not just two people speaking to each other. Facial expressions and bodily movements provide signs to other people of the way we feel. Communicating by touch is something we take for granted within our own families and something that elderly people often miss when they have been widowed or ill for a long time or have lived alone without much personal contact. Someone with dementia who has lost the gift of understanding spoken words will still be able to receive a reassuring message from the touch of a hand, an arm round the shoulders and a calm tone of voice. Continuing physical expressions of affection are just as important for those who have lost the ability to appreciate speech. This non-verbal communication can work in both directions, and the caring relative may learn a lot about the way someone is feeling by the tension and tremor in the person's hand.

Making the most of understanding

You can help to keep someone in touch with who they are, where they are and what is happening by remembering to *give information*; for example, by saying, 'It is time for lunch now, it's one o'clock', or 'This is Thursday, the day I go to collect your pension.' Be prepared to give the information two or three times and allow time for it to sink in. Try to make your conversations meaningful to the other person and use memory aids to remind her what you are talking about. Produce family photos of grandchildren when you're telling news of them. Show the headlines in the newspaper just after the news on TV or radio. Always remind someone who may forget not just the *name* of a visitor but *who* they are: 'Here's Jean, your granddaughter, come to see you', or 'It's Mrs Brown, the nurse who comes to bandage your leg.'

What other memory aids can you use? Large visible clocks, calendars, newspapers with large headlines, message boards, an essential telephone number written out near the phone – all these can be helpful, particularly for the less seriously impaired person. Don't move the furniture around more than necessary; always leave things in familiar places. You can try labelling the doors if someone had difficulty in finding the bathroom or toilet, but the lettering must be very large and clear.

Reality orientation therapy

This therapy is jokingly referred to sometimes as ROT, and sounds as if it ought to be a complicated psychological technique. In fact it is a simple approach to making the most of the memory and skills that the individual retains. The technique aims to use every opportunity of contact with the patient to remind him or her of current reality and to correct, kindly but firmly, mistaken memories. For example, when her thoughts wander back to her early life (perhaps saying, 'I'd better be getting home now. Mother will be waiting'), remind her of who she is, where she is and what she is doing at this very minute.

You can use her memory of past times very effectively to conjure up happy reminders of a life well lived. Music is a wonderful reminder. Many of us are instantly transported back to our teens by the popular songs of our own era; two bars of an Everly Brothers record and I'm straight back to my youth! Nostalgia is a pleasant emotion, and the songs and music of younger days are often happily listened to by elderly people, who may find it difficult to appreciate the music of today. The guiding principle of reality orientation is to encourage the person to understand that memories are of life in the past and to keep them in touch with what is happening here and now.

Speech problems

A dementia sufferer finds it increasingly difficult to find the right word or phrase to make others understand them. We all have such problems at times, referring to objects as 'thingamajigs' and 'what-d'you-call-its'. When this problem becomes so great that whole sentences are made up of words only approximating to what is meant, a person's speech will sound nonsensical and can give rise to problems. Instead of, 'I want a cup of tea', the words can come out as, 'Plate in the kitchen, I want to try the what's-it.' This funny-sounding mixing up of meanings, called *dysphasia*, can often be understood and translated by someone who knows the person well; but when it cannot be understood, there may be frustration and irritation on both sides. Remember that she may not be able to comprehend your normal speech either; the brain cannot translate the sounds into understandable words. As dementia progresses perhaps only one or two words or phrases will be left for her to communicate with, and it is here that your ingenuity in communicating by non-verbal expressions – facial, touch and gesture – can be so important.

Over-reacting

An individual with a failing capacity for remembering and performing ordinary tasks usually has an awareness somewhere deep inside that all is not well. It is natural to deny the frightening truth and cover up for failing powers. A person who is asked to do something that is now beyond her abilities will often react with sudden severe distress and anguish or even with tantrums of anger and frustration. This sudden outburst in the face of failure is called a *catastrophic reaction*. It can happen with something as simple as trying to lace up a shoe or turn on the television. More usually it happens on such occasions as being asked to remember a telephone message left for you or to answer questions that require a good memory. There is usually a warning moment or two of perplexed agitation before the outburst, and, with luck, you can provide a reassuring distraction.

These outbursts are not stubbornness or deliberate attempts to make life difficult for you; nor can they be stopped at will. The person can't control them. The less fuss you make the better. It is useless trying the same sort of tactics as you might try with a naughty child. A child can appreciate that he is behaving badly and reacts to his parents' anger, learning that there are more effective and socially acceptable ways of getting his own way. But someone with dementia cannot learn effectively and she may well not even remember the incident an hour or two later. Keeping calm is of course easier said than done. It may help to keep reminding yourself that this is usually a temporary phase, which the individual will eventually pass through.

In addition to the communication difficulties discussed above, the dementia sufferer and her carer may be faced with one or some of the following day-to-day problems.

Food and eating problems

Our diet is largely governed by social convention. The Japanese eat dried fish, seaweed and bean curds for breakfast – an unappetising sight for the unsuspecting foreign visitor looking forward to eggs and bacon! Similarly, the curious diets chosen by dementia sufferers often worry their relatives, who may fear that they are not getting sufficient nourishment. If your relative is living with you, however, you can easily supplement their diet with milky drinks, fresh fruit drinks or, as a last resort, vitamin supplement tablets. You can get advice from your local pharmacist on vitamin tablets.

People with dementing illnesses occasionally develop curious food fads. I know a patient who likes to eat nothing but chocolate rolls and bananas, but her family manages to persuade her to take lots of fresh orange juice and occasional food-replacement milk drinks such as Complan; she remains remarkably fit. No one needs a hot cooked meal every day to stay healthy. But although the composition of meals does not matter all that much, ideally the diet should contain sufficient roughage such as bran, wholemeal bread and fresh vegetables to prevent constipation.

The nutritional problems of patients living with a relative are not usually serious; but if you are supporting someone who lives alone, there can be a problem in ensuring that their diet is adequate. Dementia sufferers living alone frequently develop nutritional deficiencies, which can lead to a worsening of their mental faculties. If you are shopping for such a person, make sure that you buy food that needs no preparation – such as bread, cheese, cold ham, tomatoes and enriched breakfast cereals. Tinned food needs skill, dexterity and motivation to get it out of the tin and is therefore less likely to be eaten. If your relative likes only sweet biscuits (a common problem), consider buying special 'slimming biscuits' from a chemist. Paradoxically these biscuits are not only more nutritious with added iron and vitamins, they also often have more calories than ordinary biscuits. The drawback is that they are expensive compared with ordinary biscuits – but a good investment if this is all your relative will eat. The meals-on-wheels service will deliver a meal but sadly cannot necessarily supervise the eating of it. Consequently you may find stocks of aluminium containers from days back developing an unsavoury smell. If you do consider requesting meals-on-wheels, make sure you know that they will be eaten. (Preferably by the patient: the meals-on-wheels service knows full well how much it contributes to the health of Britain's cat and dog population!)

Overeating

Overeating is rare in dementia, but occasionally someone keeps asking for food just after they have finished a meal. Perhaps they cannot remember they have just eaten, or it is possible that the brain's hunger mechanism is working incorrectly. Try not to keep giving fattening foods like sweets or chocolates; a heavy person is much more difficult to care for than a light one.

Food refusal

It is normal for dementia sufferers to lose weight and to eat less as the illness progresses. This is the usual course of events and to be expected. Chewing and swallowing processes slow down because of the difficulties in co-ordinating the muscles that control swallowing, and meals may drag on for some time. The important thing is to let the individual eat at her own pace. Eventually she may refuse food altogether, and if this continues it will lead to serious malnutrition and illness, which can in turn lead to death. You must discuss this with your doctor, because it is possible that some other illness or severe depression is causing the problem. If these causes have been ruled out, one is faced with the distressing acceptance of the natural course of events. Encourage the person to take as much fluid as possible but do not force the issue. You can do more harm than good by pushing food and drink on to an unwilling frail person.

Eating habits

Table manners deteriorate in time. People with dementia may eat with the fingers, drop food, take food from other people's plates and eventually lose their skills in using utensils. Co-ordination problems may be helped by the right aids. For example, you can buy bowls with suction pads to prevent them moving on the table. When the skill to use utensils is lost, you should prepare food that can be eaten with the fingers without embarrassment. Bibs are not very dignified, but there are some attractive plastic-coated aprons that anyone can wear without looking childish.

What about alcohol?

A glass of one's favourite drink is a good appetite stimulant, a mild sedative for night-time and enjoyable; it is much tastier than a sleeping-tablet! However, if the patient is taking other medication, especially sedatives or tranquillisers, these may not mix with alcohol very well. You may find that the person becomes over-drowsy or, alternatively, more disturbed and restless at night. Alcohol is a matter of trial and error, although a moderate amount does not in general do any harm.

Washing, bathing and dressing

There are probably more heated family battles about the dementia sufferer's difficulties in this area than any other. Problems arise because the individual forgets to wash, shave or bath and loses the insight to recognise the unsavoury outcome of self-neglect. Sometimes a simple reminder is all that is required. Refusal to use the bath or shower regularly are, however, common problems. Sometimes the person hates being helped physically. An unfamiliar touch or a clumsy helping hand are difficult to tolerate if you are not used to them. Have you ever had to have a wash or bed-bath from a nurse in hospital? You will know how difficult and embarrassing it is at first until you get used to it, so it is not surprising that someone with less understanding finds it all rather threatening and unpleasant. A further reason for refusal to bath is shame over incontinence and a desire to hide the evidence. Even if you are furious and at the end of your tether (perhaps you changed her less than an hour ago), never ever blame the person for being wet and soiled; you will find a minor skirmish turning into a major battle. Like much advice in this book, I know it is much easier to give than to put into practice. Try deep breathing and let yourself calm down.

A curious phenomenon that crops up occasionally is a fear of getting in the bath or shower and of hair washing. Plenty of tact and reassurance may help. Alternatively, try a stand-up all-over wash-down instead of a bath. Remember to praise the person when she does smell nice and look smart. Compliments are appreciated by everyone.

Whenever possible, let the person dress herself. This usually takes a lot longer, and she may need some guidance and supervision. Pointing out the order clothes go on will help. Eventually the individual may need everything doing for her; but even when this is the case, as far as possible allow her to choose her own clothing for the day.

Special aids to help with bathing and dressing and special clothing are discussed in Chapter 8.

Occupation during the daytime

Left to their own devices, dementia sufferers may do nothing but sit in a chair staring into space. Alternatively, they may be very restless and spend every waking hour moving about from one room to another. This can be very wearing for the carer. There is nothing more irritating than someone jumping up and down from their chair just when you are about to have a quiet rest or watch television. The problem is, however, that a dementia sufferer has a very short attention span and needs constant stimulation and distraction. It is usually easiest to provide diversion by encouraging them to continue tasks familiar to them. Women who have knitted or done household chores all their lives often preserve these skills long after you might expect. Useful tasks such as preparing vegetables and doing the dusting may not be performed to the same standard as before but will help the person feel she still has a role to play. Men may still be able to do a little gardening, and it doesn't matter if the same spot is dug over twenty times. Introducing new hobbies and activities is more difficult. The disdain one sometimes sees on the faces of men attending day centres when they are invited to take part in painting and collage makes me think that it isn't often worth too much effort. The present generation of elderly people are not used to having much leisure time for hobbies or sport. Consequently household tasks are generally more acceptable.

Remember too to make sure that the person gets some exercise. They often remain confined to the house, scarcely moving around. A fit, mobile person is much easier to care for than an immobile, chairbound one, so try to keep them moving and if possible take them on accompanied walks and journeys outside the home. A tired patient sleeps better too.

Loss of time sense

It is common in dementia to lose track of time. A sufferer often forgets how long it is since the last meal, when to expect the next meal, when to go to bed and so on. If you go out for an hour or two leaving the person alone, it may seem to them an eternity until your return. A daytime outing away from home, to a day centre for example, can seem an interminably long separation from home. There is no easy solution to this. When you are going out, you can leave a prominent notice saying at what time you will be back. You may have to get used to a degree of temporary distress when you return. It is important not to stop going out because of this or you will soon feel trapped in the prison of your own home. You need that break.

Other common problems and peculiar habits connected with dementia include the following.

Incontinence

Incontinence means passing urine or motions in inappropriate places. Babies are incontinent because they have not yet learned to control their bladder and bowel habits. Incontinence in elderly people is very common indeed; one study found that one in three women over the age of sixty-five experiences the problem to some degree, often usually a bit of 'leakage' when coughing or laughing heartily. Women generally learn to cope very well by wearing a bit of extra protection in the form of absorbent pant-liners, for example Brevia by Kotex.

Incontinence is particularly common in dementia sufferers. There are a number of different causes, which, along with other aspects of incontinence, it is important to be aware of.

Sudden onset of incontinence of urine

Sometimes accompanied by an unpleasant smell in the urine or dark colour, such sudden incontinence may well be due to an infection in the bladder. You may also notice that the individual is more confused than usual. This is easily cured with the right antibiotic, so consult your doctor.

The toilet may be too far away to reach in time

As we age, the time betwen the sensation of wanting to pass urine and of having an urgent need to pass urine shortens. So there is no time to waste looking for where the toilet is. Finding the right place is particularly difficult for the dementia sufferer, especially when in an unfamiliar place. Make sure you rehearse with the person exactly where the toilet is and label the door. Consider having a commode by the bed if the distance is too great for safety. Men can use a bed bottle. The district nurse will advise you on bottles and commodes and will be able to loan you any equipment she judges will be useful.

Incontinence of urine may happen only at night

You can try getting up once in the night to take the person to the toilet. Alternatively, if you cannot face that, make sure the person is wearing adequate protection and that the bedding is protected. You can buy plastic mattress covers, pillowcases and large absorbent pads to place on the sheets.

A regular toilet regime

This may prove of benefit. If you take the person regularly to the toilet every two hours you may find that this avoids incontinence altogether. If the individual can hold urine for two hours you can gradually increase the time between visits to three hours or so. If you find you need to take them every hour to keep them dry, however, then the bladder is probably not capable of being trained effectively, and you probably ought to abandon toilet training and turn to protective clothing and incontinence aids.

Pads and protective clothing

These work on the same principle as disposable nappies for babies. The quality and effectiveness of these products vary widely. You can get regular supplies of pads and plastic pants through your local district nursing service but you will normally find much better, though more pricey, products through a specialist supplier. (See advice on aids, Chapter 8.) Try a comparison first; don't give up on the free products, as these are upgraded from time to time and may prove satisfactory.

Incontinence is embarrassing and distressing for the sufferer

Attempts to hide the evidence by stuffing wet pants behind a radiator or wrapping up faeces in paper or handkerchiefs and hiding the parcels in cupboards may seem bizarre and incomprehensible but they are a sign that the person is aware that she is not managing her habits correctly. She is doing her best to cope with the problem. Try to get across to her that you understand the problem and can help her tackle it.

Use of catheter

A permanent catheter is a tube into the bladder that drains off urine into a plastic bag. It is not usually a satisfactory solution for an incontinent, mobile, confused person, however. Catheters are puzzling for the patient, who often pulls out the tube, can't cope with emptying the bag and finds the whole business perplexing. Yet a bed-bound or immobile person may still find a catheter a more comfortable solution than being continually wet. Emptying a catheter bag and learning to take care of a catheter need a little skill, but a district nurse will be able to show a relative how to manage this and what to do if problems crop up.

Other causes of incontinence of urine

Besides infections in the urine, described above, other causes of incontinence are:

(1) Severe constipation.
(2) Prostate gland trouble in men. After a prostate operation, dribbling may continue for a while.
(3) 'Water tablets', i.e. diuretic drugs used to treat heart failure. These cause a sudden desire to pass a lot of urine urgently. You may be able to judge when the 'flood' is about to happen and avoid it by taking the person to the toilet at the right time.
(4) Sedatives and tranquilliser medications frequently diminish the sensation of needing to pass urine and slow down the person's motivation to get to the loo in time.
(5) Other diseases such as diabetes, stroke and bladder disease can also affect bladder control.

The district nurse is the best source of help here and she may ask the doctor to review the problem.

Incontinence of bowel motions

This form of incontinence is not common, but when it does happen it is extremely trying and unpleasant for everyone.

The usual cause of incontinence with diarrhoea is *constipation*. This may sound contradictory, but when the bowel is blocked with hard stool, leakage of fluid 'overflows' and appears as diarrhoea. A good diet rich in roughage will help to prevent it. All Bran really works!

Do not try to treat constipation with laxatives but, if it persists, consult the district nurse or doctor. The cause may be more complex and may need investigation. Regular incontinence of normally formed motions can be dealt with only by trying to judge the likely time that it will occur and taking the person to the toilet first. Otherwise you have to use the incontinence aids that are mentioned above.

Wandering

It is hard to get lost in Britain unless you're really trying to disappear. Even in Central London, where you might think elderly people could wander at will without anyone noticing, it is extremely unusual for an elderly confused person to be missing for twenty-four hours or more. The worry of losing someone for even an hour or two is nevertheless enough to start the carer's brain working overtime on possible disasters such as mugging, traffic accidents or sudden illness. Some individuals are constantly wanting to be off out of the door and can walk for miles away from home before being found. They often seem to be searching for their old home or looking for a long-dead relative. This kind of wandering is common after a move into a new home or into a nursing home.

There are two sensible precautions you can take if your relative is a persistent 'wanderer'. First, fit a lock on the outside doors that cannot be opened easily by an unskilled person and fit extra locks at the bottom and top of doors. Second, make sure that name, address and your phone number are attached to the person somewhere. An identity bracelet is invaluable. Some individuals become agitated and resentful when prevented from pursuing their adventure, however; in such instances, rather than confronting them and trying to prevent it, the best approach is to walk along with them and steer them home or divert them into some other activity.

When someone disappears it is likely that you will feel guilty and that you should have been taking better notice. You may feel that other people will blame you. Usually, in fact, the carer blames him- or herself considerably more than others do. People recognise that it is a superhuman feat to keep a person in your sights all the time. Unfortunately, day centres and old people's homes often share these concerns and may not welcome wanderers because of the staff's anxiety about losing someone. They worry that disaster will strike and that they will be blamed by relatives and by their own managers. (Also, the local press may well make an issue out of someone wandering off and may therefore be insensitive in its reporting of an event.) The best way of dealing with this is for the relatives of the patient to reassure the centre or home that they won't think it is their fault if the person goes missing on the odd occasion.

You may think that this is being a little dismissive of the problem, but little harm usually comes to a wanderer. Someone with a lot of energy needs an outlet for it. Plenty of accompanied walks and outings may prove useful substitutes; but in any event *there is no medication that prevents wandering*. Doses of tranquillising medication sufficient to prevent wandering will make the individual drowsy, more confused and often incontinent. This is never the answer to the problem.

Disturbance at night

As mentioned already, dementia impairs the sense of time. It is common for the sufferer to be quite docile and acquiescent during the day but overactive, wide awake and raring to be out of the house at night. It is not uncommon for such people to set off to do the shopping or pick up the pension at three o'clock in the morning, unable to distinguish night from day. Everyone is kept awake by a restless person padding about the house in a confused state. A carer with the steadiest nerves can be sorely tried by nights of lying awake, nervously waiting for the sound of a fall. If the individual is well and truly tired out by a day of physical activity she is likely to sleep better at night; conversely, if she is slumped in front of a TV in and out of sleep all day, it is scarcely surprising if she is 'on the go' all night. So keep her as active as possible during the day. If the problem persists night after night, ask the doctor about whether a night sedative might help; if severe night disturbance goes on for too long *you'll* end up needing the sedatives, so deal with the problem early on.

Odd ideas and beliefs

'This isn't my home. I want to go to my own home'

The ability to recognise a familiar room or house may be lost in dementia. The room appears perplexingly different, and the sufferer may be convinced that she is being held against her will in a strange place. A person may refuse to enter the house or sit outside for hours waiting to be 'taken home'. Try in these circumstances to point out familiar items of furniture, mementoes and photographs that might be recognised. These sometimes trigger off recognition. Bear in mind how frightened the individual feels about being lost in an unfamiliar place, and respond accordingly with plenty of verbal reassurance.

'I don't know you. You aren't my daughter'

A sufferer's closest relative, who is with the person day in and day out, may suddenly be accused of being a different person, a substitute for the loved one or a stranger. The underlying problem is the failing brain's inability to recognise faces. This is not necessarily associated with a poor memory and may be an isolated symptom. Because the individual may be able to remember that she is cared for by her daughter or husband, for example, it is a terrifying experience for her to feel abandoned to a stranger whose face she cannot recognise. If you are the caring relative you will find this rejection hurtful and distressing. You won't be able to argue or persuade her but you must try to keep reassuring her. Sometimes another familiar face can be recognised, so try summoning another helping relative to reassure her.

'Someone's been stealing from me'; 'My belongings are missing'; 'Someone's been rearranging my room'

Suspicious ideas that people are stealing things, trying to harm them and plotting against them are forms of *paranoia* (see Chapter 10). We have all misplaced objects and forgotten where we put them and at times we may wonder whether the objects have been stolen. However, we do not worry seriously whether misplaced spectacles have been stolen or whether our half-used tablets of soap have been taken, since reason tells us that no one would want them. But dementia sufferers lose objects easily and are unable to reason sensibly to reassure themselves. Imagine how difficult it is to keep track of where you put things when your memory can hold information for only a moment or two.

Some people seem naturally to be more suspicious than others, to take against people more easily and to be over-sensitive to imagined slights. These personality traits may be exaggerated by the perplexing experience of dementia. Instead of contradicting paranoid ideas, try searching for the lost object or give some reassurance that you know where the missing things are.

When a suspicious idea solidifies into a peculiar fixed belief that time and argument do not diminish, we refer to the belief as a *delusion*. For example, a man with dementia became convinced that the neighbours were spying on him and sat all day in the dark behind closed curtains 'to prevent them looking in'. He began to believe his food was poisoned and stopped eating the meals delivered to him. Eventually he went into a nursing home and then began to accuse his daughters of stealing all his money. He could not comprehend their explanation that his money was being used to pay for his nursing care and had forgotten their earlier explanations. Persistent delusional ideas can sometimes be helped by specific medication.

'You're trying to get rid of me'; 'You want me to go into a home'

However ill-founded in reality these notions may be, they are highly distressing for the sufferer. They are also embarrassing for the carers and can provoke guilty feelings. Chapter 4 discusses these upsetting, ambivalent feelings in greater depth. The fear of abandonment and loss of affection that these ideas express can be helped only by constant reassurance and genuine signs of affection and warmth.

You cannot easily cheat here. You may imagine that what is being discussed in private with the rest of the family does not sink in, but the person is often very sensitive to atmosphere and tension. They know they are a burden and are creating a lot of trouble for you and others. Constant reassurance is worth giving if you really do feel committed. It is important to express your warm feelings, but also you should be truthful about your future plans. If you are considering a placement in a nursing home you must involve the individual at an early stage. Chapter 6 discusses how and when to decide on nursing home care.

Difficult behaviour

The smaller irritations caused by a dementia sufferer's odd behaviour may sometimes be the 'straw that breaks the camel's back' for the relative. The most frequent problems are a constant repetition of the same questions throughout the day, a tendency to follow close relatives around, clinging and forbidding the person to be out of sight even for a minute or two, an inability to sit still and continuous restless pacing around. In a small flat or house these problems can seem much, much worse than they really are.

The annoyance and upset you will naturally feel can wear you down if you do not learn to ignore this behaviour or at least get a regular break from the person's presence. Losing your temper will raise their anxiety level further and is unlikely to be effective in stopping the problem behaviour. So try to keep your temper under control, however hard this may be. Remember to think through the reasons for the odd behaviour. The search for reassurance from a trusted person is one of the few sources of security for a dementia sufferer.

With some patients there is a more complex reason for the behaviour, however. Brain damage can 'waken up' parts of the brain so that it becomes more alert than usual, causing the person to pace restlessly, aimlessly and continuously. They are driven by an uncontrollable urge to keep on the move the whole time. This problem can sometimes be helped by medication but it requires very careful monitoring because of the risk of making the person drowsy, fall over or become more confused. Some medication can even be the primary cause of this restless urge to be on the go, so great care is needed in assessing the effect of medication to make sure that it does not make the problem worse.

Aggressiveness

There are three main types of problem that fall under this heading. The first sort of aggressiveness, manifested by frequent use of abusive language, outbursts of temper and sudden thoughtless lashing out, can be due to the exaggeration of former personality traits. A moody, bad-tempered, bossy sergeant-major type who has been inclined in his younger days to flare up and bash his wife is unlikely to become all sweetness and smiles as his brain begins to fail. A man with poor control of his temper will usually have even poorer control when he develops dementia. You will notice I say 'he' rather than 'she' because, on the whole, it is men who have lifelong problems with controlling their tempers to the point where they become physically violent to their families. Women have developed different responses to frustrating situations. They tend to become depressed and anxious, whereas men are more inclined to respond to frustration with anger and violence.

The second sort of aggressiveness is caused by fright and despair. Most commonly, the person does not recognise who is looking after them and lashes out instinctively. This behaviour was mentioned earlier in the section on bathing and hygiene. Some people hate to be touched by others and dislike the close contact that is necessitated by being dependent on others for care. If you take a lot of trouble to explain exactly what you are going to do and why, and allow time for the person to take it in, most people will eventually tolerate what needs to be done, especially if the hands are soothing and gentle.

The third sort of aggressiveness is probably the most frightening for the carer but thankfully is extremely unusual. Here the individual becomes unpredictably destructive and violent for no apparent reason. This violence may not necessarily be accompanied by anger or loss of temper and usually takes the form of a sudden, thoughtless, unpremeditated punch or pinch. It is unpleasant and hurtful but it is entirely without spite; dementia prevents the person from being either 'plotting' or spiteful.

How should you cope with physical aggression? Rule one: never hit back 'to teach him a lesson'. He cannot learn the lesson, and we know that the harsher any human being is treated the more likely he is to respond with more aggression. Hitting back may well make the problem worse. Rule two: get out of the way; don't try to restrain someone. Rule three: get help – from a relative, friend, neighbour or anyone who is sensible and calm. Above all, remember that you cannot 'blame' the patient.

Sexual behaviour

People with dementia may continue to have quite normal sexual drives. They may however begin to behave in an uninhibited way in public because their brain damage has weakened their control and made them forget what is socially appropriate. A man may consequently stroke his genitals in public without realising the embarrassment this causes to others. Don't worry that the person is becoming 'over-sexed'; they are not. This is a normal human activity, particularly in men; so just remind him tactfully where he is and why it is not considered polite to do it here.

Some men with dementia, however, sometimes make excessive sexual demands on their wives. It can be very wearing for the wife to be sexually approached every few hours, particularly when she may have lost her sexual desire for him a long time ago, possibly as a result of the illness. If the situation seems to be getting out of hand and you really cannot manage to dissuade him with tact then you could consult your doctor about medications that can help to damp down an excessive sex drive.

One further point about sex: it is quite normal for couples to continue to have intercourse even when one spouse has early dementia. The caring spouse may find that the person needs more help and guidance than before, but no one should feel guilty about continuing to express affection in this way.

Mood problems and depression

Anger, fear, moodiness, anxiety and perplexed puzzlement are all understandable emotions in a dementing person, particularly at the beginning of the illness when the individual has some partial awareness of her failing capacities. Often with time this gives way to a mood of 'emptiness' accompanied by a bland passive acceptance. Some unfortunate sufferers develop severe distress and are continuously tearful, agitated and fearful, as if marooned on an isolated island without help. It is difficult to reassure these people that they are being cared for, and this is very painful for the carer to watch, unable to help.

Depression, however, is rather different (see Chapter 9). If people with dementia become low and depressed, they cannot express their sadness in words very easily. Instead they often become slow and withdrawn and appear more confused and forgetful. Their appetite is poor, and they lose weight. They may make remarks about feeling wicked or may believe themselves to be physically ill. When someone has dementia, it is notoriously difficult to decide if there is depression there too. If you are worried that your relative may have depression as well as dementia, ask the doctor to assess her again as it may be possible to improve the patient's mood.

Sudden changes of mood

Sudden outbursts of tears for no apparent reason or for an inappropriate and trivial reason, for example, often occur after a major stroke or in individuals with multi-infarct dementia. This is frequently combined with a distressing tendency to burst out laughing inappropriately. This 'emotional lability' is easily confused with depression. The clue to establishing the right cause is that true depression is a *persistent* feeling of sadness that the person cannot be 'jollied' out of temporarily.

Hallucinations (visions and voices)

Dementia sufferers often complain of 'seeing things'. Seeing things that are not really there, usually people, children, animals or insects, is a frightening experience. You must realise that the objects appear to the person as real and solid for a while, so it is not helpful for you to respond with, 'It's just your imagination.' On the other hand you should not collude with the person either. Reassure them that you understand how frightening the experience is, but do not imply that you can see the vision too. Visual hallucinations usually occur in people with poor sight; 'flashing lights' and 'disco lights' occur often in people with glaucoma. Have the individual's eyes checked by a specialist. Ensure that the lighting is adequate in the rooms in the evening, so that there is less likelihood of misinterpretation of objects around. If they persist or become serious, hallucinations can be treated with the right medication, so you should consult your doctor. If your relative persistently hears voices you should similarly seek a medical opinion.

There are in addition some unusual perceptual experiences that are connected with a 'failure to recognise' problem. A person may, for example, believe that the image in a mirror is somebody else. This is less of a problem when the mirror image is assumed to be a friend, but it may be seen as an enemy. A parallel is that the image of a person on television or in a photograph may be treated as a real person in the room.

Sensible safety precautions and guarding against risk

You cannot wrap up the sufferer in cotton wool and watch her every minute of the day. It is not fair to the individual to curtail physical movements or daily activities too much. Falls, fractures and minor accidents will happen, and it is better to allow a little more freedom than you are really comfortable with, even if you know it entails some risk, than be too smothering and protective. You can nevertheless take some practical measures to reduce the risk of accidents.

(1) *Go over the house and remove all obstacles*, such as loose rugs, loose bits of worn carpet, wiring, telephone cables, ornaments and anything that someone could trip over easily. Tack down the stair carpet. Parquet and highly polished vinyl floors are like skating-rinks, so cover them up or stop polishing them.

(2) *Throw away those old slippers* with flattened backs that are

so easy to trip over. Invest in some comfortable supporting slippers.

(3) *Do not economise on light bulbs.* Forty-watt bulbs are inadequate. Put good lighting in all the rooms your relative uses, especially in the bedroom, bathroom, on the landing and on the stairs.

(4) *Check whether you need handrails* on the stairs or in the bathroom. See Chapter 8, the section on aids, for details.

(5) *Gas stoves and gas fires* are difficult to light and dangerous if turned on and left unlit. A person with dementia living alone should not be left to use gas appliances unsupervised. Electric kettles should have an automatic cut-out to prevent them boiling dry.

(6) In the case of a person living alone, *consider how the home is heated.* Dementia sufferers do not feel the cold as sharply as usual and are more likely to forget to turn on the heating. It is essential to have the home permanently heated during a British winter. Automatically controlled storage heaters and central heating systems that can be controlled by relatives or neighbours are far better than appliances that the person has to turn on and off personally. If you have to have open fires, make sure they have guards.

(7) *Put medicines in a locked cupboard* or out of sight. Do not expect the patient to take medicine without supervision.

(8) *Have secure locks fitted* to the outer doors but ensure that there are duplicate keys. Remove any internal door-chains, which may prevent access in an emergency.

(9) *Alarm call systems* are systems where there is a telephone link to a special number so that a disabled person can get help in an emergency. They are *not* designed for the confused elderly. People have to be alert to press the button or pull the cord at the right time. Dementia sufferers either ignore the system because they do not know when they need assistance or press the button frequently and unnecessarily, generating much anxiety and irritation.

(10) *Do not let your relative drive* under any circumstances. If necessary, remove the car keys.

4

Dementia: How the Carer Feels

Caring for a person with dementia is one of the most difficult jobs anyone can undertake. It is both emotionally and physically draining. The caring person is often surprised and worried by their own strong reactions towards the patient and also towards other relatives. At some stage most carers feel isolated, unsupported, discouraged and unhappy. These feelings then engender guilt, anxiety and tension, and this can be almost overwhelming. Human beings vary enormously in their ability to approach such problems phlegmatically. Some of us are born worriers and are constantly brooding pessimistically about possible catastrophes. Others are of a more optimistic, calm nature, and take difficulties in their stride. One thing is certain: you cannot change yourself. So this chapter describes some of the common feelings that carers talk about, aiming to give reassurance that these feelings are normal and understandable. The discussion then turns to how other people can help and support you while you are coping with the problem.

Grief

The experience of grief can follow any permanent major loss in our lives and is not confined to the period after the death of someone close. When a husband or wife dies, the bereaved person goes through a time of profound sadness with feelings of yearning to have the lost person back again, episodes of despairing tearfulness and a fatiguing feeling of being panicky and 'keyed up' without any obvious cause.

When a close relative develops dementia, particularly a husband or wife, the loved person slowly slips away from the relationship as a result of the illness and can no longer provide the companionship and mutual caring that characterised the relationship before the illness. As dementia deepens, the caring spouse is in fact being bereaved in the cruellest way. This leads to grief, and such feelings are even harder to bear than ordinary grief because they drag on for the duration of the illness and cannot be properly resolved until the affected person dies. It is only then that time slowly starts to heal the loss and the bereaved person can begin to remember with love the real person they married so long ago.

Feelings of grief, sadness and longing for the past are therefore all normal in someone caring for a loved one suffering from dementia. These feelings are often interspersed with bursts of hopefulness and optimism that the person will recover, that a cure will be found or that they will improve a little. As time goes on, however, the carer usually accepts the inevitable fact of the sufferer's decline.

Relatives, friends and neighbours rally round after a death to give support and comfort to a bereaved person; but a carer's grief is often invisible. Other people may fail to understand how distressed the carer has become.

It can be so painful watching someone suffer from dementia that sometimes the carer feels that they wish the sufferer dead: 'I cannot bear it any longer. I just want this terrible illness to be over. I want him to die quickly to end his suffering.' This is an extremely common but bewildering feeling. When you love someone it seems inconceivable that you should wish the person dead. Carers sometimes query whether their prayers to have the illness over really reflect their own inability to tolerate the distress. Are such feelings due to selfishness or love? Such questions often lead the carer to feel guilty. But the wish for death to come quickly to a loved person in distress partly reflects an acceptance that the old relationship is over, that the sufferer can never be the same person and that the proper grieving that follows loss can happen only when the person finally dies.

Anger

The repetitive symptoms of dementia are extremely irritating. Such things as constant questioning, following you around and doing silly things without thought can be infuriating to those whose best efforts to care seem thwarted by the patient. A daughter caring for her demented father said:

> He hates being wet. He's always been very fastidious, so we go to the bathroom more or less every hour. What really drives me crazy is that the minute we're in the bathroom he won't wait to get his clothes off properly. He gets into a terrible panic, fumbles furiously with his clothes and usually floods every-where, so there's always a major cleaning job. It happens every time. I found myself yelling at him to slow down as if he could help it. I really let go, called him silly and stupid and said he was doing it deliberately. The minute I calmed down I felt awful; upset and guilty. He can't help it, I know. But if only he'd let me help him!

Feeling cross and shouting at the person are understandable but not usually helpful. Expressing anger in shouting abuse often makes the sufferer's behaviour worse. They sense the tension and frustration and begin to behave in an agitated, anxious way. This can lead to a vicious circle of rising tension and explosive behaviour on both sides.

'She does it to upset me.' The feeling that the individual has singled out the carer for her most difficult behaviour is understandable when the person appears to behave per-fectly in the company of others, especially strangers:

She's on the move all day, up and down, round the
house, just won't sit still. It works me up till I can
scream at her. And at the day centre she just sits
calmly with the others at one table. She even joins in
the activities there and is helping to make a picture.
They don't believe me when I tell them what she is like
at home, she's so placid and co-operative there.

This daughter felt as if her mother somehow had her singled
out personally to upset her; she felt her mother was trying
to get her own back on her for times in the past when the
daughter herself had been a rebellious teenager. It was
difficult for this daughter to understand that sufferers can
and do behave very differently in different environments. A
person with dementia rarely behaves consciously in a
difficult or annoying way; to do this would require a
motivation that they no longer possess. Dementia sufferers
do not deliberately give up household tasks or activities
until they cannot perform them or concentrate adequately.
*The feeling of relatives that the person could do more for themselves
if they tried is almost always wrong*. Getting cross with them
and trying to bully them into performing better is doomed to
failure.

Venting your anger verbally on the individual will upset
both of you but will do no permanent harm. The danger
comes when you find yourself expressing frustration and
anger physically. A son-in-law described what happened
one evening:

She keeps going to put the kettle on and then leaves it,
comes back to sit down and forgets about it. We've
burnt four kettles already. This time my wife was out
and I was in the garden. I saw her filling the kettle and
turning on the ring through the window. I shouted to
her to watch it and then got on with my work. Sure
enough, a few minutes later I smelt burning, saw
smoke coming out and ran into the kitchen and found
two tea towels had been left on top of the stove and
were alight! Another minute and the house would
have been in flames. Mother was calmly watching. I

> grabbed her and shook her, shouting at her. I shoved
> her against a wall and she fell over. It was only when I
> saw she couldn't get up by herself that I realised what
> I'd done. The next day her arms were covered in black
> bruises where I'd grabbed her – she bruises so easily.

Shaking, shoving and feeling murderous towards the elderly person are danger signals that you *must* get help. Whether you need a temporary or a permanent break from the person you are caring for, you must discuss what is happening with a doctor, a social worker, your clergyman, a relative or friend you trust, *someone*. Violent incidents are a sign that you are not coping. They tend to recur even when you swear to yourself that it will never happen again. Physical harm usually occurs where desperate but loving and caring relatives are at the end of their tether and lash out in anger during a frustrating incident.

Professionals occasionally come across tragic cases where one member of the family regularly physically abuses an elderly relative; often it is a son or son-in-law, who drinks heavily and has long-standing difficulties managing his life even without the added strain of a dependent elderly person in the house. But this kind of 'granny battering' is rare.

Guilt

When you, the carer, feel angry with someone you love who has developed dementia, this gives rise to feelings of guilt and shame. This is especially true if the anger and irritation have led to thoughtless or selfish behaviour towards the sufferer.

Guilt can be a useful emotion for human beings. It is the feeling that motivates us to do what we perceive to be our duty towards our family, workmates and friends even when we would rather be doing something else. It is the feeling that tells us we have not done enough and have failed to achieve the high standards of conduct we have set for ourselves.

Unfortunately, guilt is a feeling that has a long memory, and the reasons why we feel guilty towards a particular person are often lost in the mists of our childhood. As we look back to our childhood days there is often one member of our close family, a parent or a brother or sister, towards whom we feel some unresolved guilt about our relationship with them. We feel that we have failed them in some way. This 'normal' guilt, which we all have in some degree towards those close to us, can sometimes surface again when in later life a carer has to look after the person they felt guilty towards. Unpleasant feelings have a habit of rising to the surface. Such guilt is particularly hard to deal with if the caring person never grew to like the person who is now suffering from dementia and needs care. In this situation, children often find themselves going overboard to do the right thing for a dementing parent, spurred on by a sense of duty. But the unpleasant feelings of guilt may well be compounded by a feeling of distaste or even hatred towards the dementing person.

Another kind of guilt may be felt by relatives who have placed an elderly person in residential care, knowing that the care their relative is receiving is impersonal and worse than the family could have given if they had been willing to do so. Such feelings of having let down the loved one, of being too weak and incapable of managing, may be made worse by the reproaches of the confused person, who cannot comprehend what a burden she has become. A daughter described her feelings like this:

> My mother was one of those Cockney marvels. She brought up my brother and me single handed by scrubbing and cleaning other people's houses all day and half the night to keep us together as a family. My dad died of flu when he came back from the First World War, and of course I never knew him. And now she needs us, we've just not been able to help. There's only me to look after her, and my husband says there's no way he could stand having her to live with us, even if we did have room, because they've never got on. So

she's in a home now and I can't bear the way she looks at me. 'Take me home with you, luv,' she keeps repeating. It's breaking my heart, feeling I've let her down.

The most important way to handle guilt is to *recognise* the way you feel and make sure you do not over-react to it by committing yourself to a more caring role than you can handle due to an overwhelming sense of duty. Realise that you are not a saint, that no one expects you to be and that you may be justified in making a selfish choice in order to look after your own needs and wishes and those of the rest of your family. Realise too that you cannot make everything come right for the elderly person. You did not bring on the dementia and it is no good blaming yourself for it. Nor can you make up to the individual for the tragedy that is happening to her.

Shame and embarrassment

Relatives are often worried that their dementia sufferer's behaviour will be misunderstood and disapproved of by strangers. People can of course be rude, staring and intolerant, but on the whole the general public is remarkably understanding. Dementia sufferers do behave in an embarrassing way sometimes, making rude remarks to strangers, blatantly and untruthfully complaining of ill-treatment to visitors, passing urine in inappropriate places, talking loudly in public places or meetings where a hushed voice or whisper is more appropriate. Their eating habits can be embarrassingly sloppy too. The sense of shame decreases as the family get used to it. You can help to minimise the embarrassment to others by explaining the illness and its effects to neighbours and relatives. They will nearly always understand and often are pleased to offer help of some kind. So try not to be shy about the problem with neighbours and strangers.

You may also find that you look back at embarrassing

moments as something to laugh about. I well remember a patient of mine, a retired nurse with a reputation for being a strict disciplinarian in her time, eyeing a group of local dignitaries who were visiting the hospital ward where she was a patient. She prodded one of the gentlemen in the back and remarked, 'Your shoes are dirty and your collar's frayed. Disgraceful, coming out like that.' We were accustomed to this patient's forthright and sometimes rude observations and so ignored her comment – at least until we saw a red flush of embarrassment creep over the visitor's face! After all, she had been right. The ward staff laugh about it now, but it was an awkward moment at the time.

Problems in the family

Taking on a new role

When we are children we depend on our parents and, on the whole, follow their wishes, looking to them for guidance and emotional support. At this stage, parents are clearly 'in charge'. As we grow through the transitional period of adolescence to adulthood our relationship with our parents changes, so that eventually we have a more equal adult relationship. The relationship can never be completely equal as we do not totally lose our feelings of being our parents' children; we still tend to bow to their wishes, even when we have established families of our own and have new responsibilities. As parents age, the role of parent and adult child begins to change once again. Young people confide less in their aged parents about their personal problems, whereas elderly people often begin to feel more like confiding their problems to their children than they have previously. It is natural, in other words, for elderly parents, particularly those who have become widowed, to begin to depend a little on their children for practical and emotional support. There is a natural 'role reversal', the parent now taking a more dependent role and the children the more sheltering, protective role.

When a parent develops dementia he or she becomes heavily dependent on others for care. Most people in this situation find it easier to depend on their own children and become 'like children', reversing the roles of earlier years, than to rely on professional carers. These natural patterns of relationship do not hold for all families, however. In many families a parent with a dominant, strong personality remains 'in charge' even when elderly and dependent. The children continue to behave towards this ageing parent in an acquiescent and subservient way even when they have become responsible for them, putting the parent's wishes before those of their own family.

Most of us know of grown-up 'mummy's boys' who have never been able to break away from the influence of a tyrannical mother and make lives of their own; or of daughters who have been 'tied to their mother's apron strings', unwilling to challenge the parent's supremacy. When these strong-willed parents suffer dementia, the subservient adult children find themselves in the painful situation of having to mature very fast in order to establish more control so that they can provide effective care for the dementia sufferer. Occasionally they seem unable to muster the strength to resist the parent's demands. They carry on treating the person as if he or she were still capable of exerting the same control over them. For example, they are unable to drum up the courage to tell a dementing parent that she needs help, that she must go to hospital for a check-up or that she must go to a day centre.

Physical care tasks such as bathing and changing are especially hard for children to perform when they have not yet come to terms with the change in the dementia sufferer.

A similar problem sometimes crops up between husband and wife where one partner has been the dominant, controlling one. Difficulties arise when the strong spouse becomes dependent on the formerly weaker half. The weaker person has then to begin to make decisions for the dementia sufferer. This is a difficult skill to acquire for someone used to depending on another person. Learning new practical skills is easier than learning to make decisions and learning to take responsibility for planning the future.

The weaker spouse has difficulty in asserting himself firmly in managing the sufferer's behaviour, especially if he is used to a lifetime of saying 'yes' to keep the peace in the marital home. Visitors to such a household often find it hard to understand why a husband or wife is not able to be firmer with the spouse – for example, in insisting that the patient attend a day hospital, in leaving her with a sitter or in allowing a GP to visit.

If being 'too weak' is your problem, consider carefully your previous relationship with the dementia sufferer. Are you reluctant to acknowledge that the relationship must change? Are you making life harder for yourself and the patient by not 'taking the bull by the horns'? Try making a small decision first and stick to it; you will then find that the larger decisions eventually become easier. A sense of mastery and maturity is achieved only with practice.

Putting the sufferer before the family

When someone becomes worn out with the care of an elderly person, everyone else in the family suffers too. A wife who is constantly fatigued, worried and anxious, or who spends a great part of her time devoting physical care to an elderly parent, often forgets that she is neglecting her own husband and family. It is very hard to be objective about the strain imposed on the rest of the family, and often the carer feels caught between two opposing sets of responsibilities. On the one hand she feels a duty towards the elderly person and feels she cannot let the person suffer; on the other hand she knows it is not fair to her husband to let the burden interfere so much with their lives. There is no doubt that many heated arguments between spouses are about responsibilities to the elderly. These become very painful when the spouse has always made it clear that he did not much like his in-laws and would have preferred to see much less of them even before the dementia began. The caring spouse then retaliates by accusing her husband of thoughtlessness and lack of feeling, thus making matters worse.

If you and your spouse are usually close and have a good marriage, heed the warning signs when you start to row over a parent. Get your priorities right and decide what is best to secure a happy future for yourselves. Some people choose to sacrifice their marriage for the care of an elderly parent because sometimes past loyalties can seem to exert stronger ties than the marriage. The penalty for this can be a lifetime of regret after the elderly person dies. On the other hand, I have known people who used their elderly parent's illness as an excuse for leaving an unsatisfactory marriage. Folks have different motives for doing what they do. Try to look objectively at the motives that lie behind the decisions you make.

'There are others who could help. Why does it all fall on me?'

Some lucky people manage to have several equally caring, equally devoted children who all get on together, but this is extremely rare. I remember meeting an Italian family who were so well organised that all seven children took an equal share in the burden of caring for their demented mother. The timetabling and organisation of the rest of their family lives needed the kind of 'flexible rostering' system that British Rail would envy. Usually, however, the major burden falls on one child, and often this child receives little help from brothers and sisters. This is sometimes due to sheer thoughtlessness on the other children's part, to a lack of awareness of how stressful it is having day-to-day care of a person with dementia. There may be other problems too. For example, the husband or wife of an unhelpful sibling may not be willing to get involved or be responsible and may put a great deal of pressure on the other partner to 'steer well clear'. Alternatively, the unsupportive children may have other pressing problems that take precedence; financial, health, marital or family difficulties of their own may preoccupy them.

Families have traditional ways of dividing up their respons-ibilities, and one member often does all the organising and takes responsibility for getting things done. It is usually daughters and daughters-in-law rather than the male members of a family who seem to get saddled with the difficult caring roles. This is partly because traditionally women are the caring, nurturing sex who take on the physical child-rearing tasks as a matter of course and are used to being good nurses. Also, they have in the past frequently not been employed outside the home and therefore are available for taking on care tasks at home. Times change, and nowadays a family may well be economically dependent on a woman's earnings. Nevertheless, women still adopt the stereotyped caring role that society has traditionally expected of them. If there is a problem in this area, try to discuss frankly with your brothers and sisters what help you need. Do not wait for them to offer help but ask for it in a straightforward way. You may be pleasantly surprised by their response. If they cannot help you, try not to let their failing cause a permanent rift between you. They may be less able to cope than you are, for a variety of reasons. In the future they might change their minds.

'I don't want to burden the children. They've got their own lives to lead'

Married couples are used to sharing problems together and often pride themselves on not involving their grown-up children in their difficulties. Busy young adults with small children often do have a lot on their minds, but an elderly parent who needs help in managing a spouse with dementia should not try to hide the problems from the adult children. Sooner or later the children will find out anyway and may feel hurt that they have been excluded from the family burden. Children want to take their share in the responsibilities, knowing that they are giving a little relief to the main carer.

Carers often feel too that they cannot go and stay even for a few days with their grown-up children or with other relatives for fear of exposing them to the tragedy: 'My daughter leads such a busy life, with her husband and children and her job. I couldn't possibly burden her with my husband for a weekend. It is so exhausting, watching him all the time. It would ruin their weekend. I'd rather not worry them.' The daughter in this family could not offer much help on a day-to-day basis but was willing to have her dementing father for regular weekends. Her mother would not accept this offer, leaving the daughter feeling cross, frustrated and extremely worried about the increasing strain on her mother. The moral here is *let other people help*. Accepting help with graciousness is a skill that has to be practised.

The need to talk to someone

Confiding our problems and joys to someone close is a very important human need. 'Getting things off your chest' can be a relief in itself. By talking things through with a person outside the situation it is often possible to find a completely different perspective on a problem; alternative options can be properly appraised when someone valued gives their views on a problem. Caring for someone with dementia can be a very lonely business indeed, and it really does help to talk to someone else about what is happening. If your husband or wife is the sufferer, it can be difficult at first to confide in someone else, but you will almost certainly find that other relatives and friends are understanding, given the chance. In Chapter 5 we consider some of the professional workers who are often prepared to act as listeners and counsellors.

Support groups

'I've got enough on my mind without talking endlessly about the problems'; 'Talking about problems doesn't make them go away'; 'Coping with my own difficulties is bad enough. I couldn't bear to hear about other people's too.' These are some of the initial reactions one hears to the suggestion that attending a regular weekly support group for relatives may help someone trying to cope with a person with dementia. These are natural reactions. People who become regular attenders and find the group most helpful usually come initially out of curiosity, because they've been bullied into it by someone or because it seems a way of keeping a link to a service that might be needed if the situation gets worse.

The aim of a support group is to provide a regular meeting of people who are all in the same boat – that is, who are the main source of support and care for a person with dementia. Groups take many forms. Sometimes they provide just an opportunity to meet, have a cup of tea, share experiences and swap information about local facilities. Other groups invite professionals to speak on topics of relevance – for example, the local psychogeriatrician, a specialist social worker or an occupational therapist. Most relatives find the groups helpful. They discover that the funny things their own relative gets up to are common, that odd, bizarre habits are quite usual and that other people have somehow coped. Some carers find to their surprise that they can give worthwhile advice to others, having become experts without realising it.

There are support groups all over Britain. Some are organised by the statutory services, but most are organised by volunteer and self-help groups. The Alzheimer's Disease Society is a rapidly growing organisation that provides a counselling service and runs many carers' groups. Age Concern and MIND also run such groups. Local churches too are active in this field. Many groups provide facilities so that you can take your relative along with you, to be looked after by someone else while you talk and relax. Other groups provide a sitting service, so you do not have to fret about what is happening at home. *If there is a group in your area, make an effort to go along*, even if you are sceptical about its value. If there is no group in your area, you might consider starting one. All you need is one or two other families or carers and perhaps a helpful professional person to get you started. Addresses to contact are listed in the Appendix.

Taking a break

A future of monotonous, never-ending caring without a break creates a sense of despair, of being trapped in a hopeless, endless process of hard work and worry. If you can look forward to a break, however, if only for a few hours or days, this can make the task much more tolerable. There is suddenly something to look forward to.

It is essential for everyone to acknowledge their need for a break. Carers often struggle on, refusing offered breaks because they feel they can manage for the moment. They frequently have a vague feeling in the back of their mind that what is being offered is not worth pursuing because it is not a total solution, or they may feel guilty about taking a short break. The practical ways of taking a break for short and long periods are covered in Chapter 5.

Are there any rewards for carrying on caring?

People rightfully feel proud of fulfilling their responsibilities with honour. There is no doubt that those who care for their relatives at home for a long time often acquire a reassuring self-knowledge that they have been tested to the limit and have come through the ordeal knowing that somehow they coped. A commitment discharged satisfactorily can leave behind it the good feeling that you did your best and are a stronger person as a result of it. Even the stress and problems of day-to-day care may not be all bad. After all, many elderly dependants are able to express their affection and gratitude in their own way and can provide a very real reward for a relative's labours.

Dementia is nevertheless probably one of the most stressful illnesses in its effect on caring relatives. The most appropriate way of tackling the personal stress is, first, by recognising and facing up to the emotional turmoil and, second, by taking steps to minimise the stress by getting practical help, regular breaks and someone to confide in.

5

Dementia: Sources of Practical Help

If you are a relative of a person with dementia, you will have already discovered that the government's slogan for the elderly of 'care in the community' means care by *you*, the relative. This being the case, how can you muster the help you need?

A bewildering variety of community services exists in Britain, but their availability is unevenly distributed. It is often a matter of luck what you will find in your own area. Services have developed on an *ad hoc* basis, usually with little co-ordination between them. Co-operation between services may be made more difficult by professional 'demarcation disputes'. For example, a home help may not wish to take responsibility for supervising tablets, which means that a district nurse may call for this one task. There is insufficient flexibility, which can mean one elderly person having up to six callers in the same day to give help that could have been provided by one person. This often leads to the elderly person receiving too little help from each service. The dilemma for the organisers of services is whether to spread themselves thinly and give a little bit of time to all those who qualify for the service or whether to concentrate their efforts on the most needy. The usual decision is to spread the service thinly; and so no one gets sufficient help, although everyone can get a little.

Planning a package of services for your relative

The most important first step is to find out what is available in your area. The four sources of help are (1) district health authority services, (2) local authority services (together referred to as 'the statutory services'), (3) voluntary organisations and (4) private services that you can buy.

'I'm all right. I don't need any help'

Before considering what you can reasonably expect from these various services, there is one sticky problem that you may have to face. The elderly person with dementia often feels fine and has no insight at all into her inability to manage by herself. She doesn't see the dirt or recognise that her home is cold and chaotic. Moreover, women who have always prided themselves on doing all their own housework and cooking can find it irksome to have someone else around doing such work. The offer of help is therefore often rejected out of hand. Similarly, it may be difficult to persuade someone that they need to visit a doctor. After all, any one of us would think it odd if our relatives kept pushing us to go to the doctor when we felt perfectly well. But don't give up trying to put in services at the first refusal. Try to persuade the visiting service to call several times just to have a chat, to gain her confidence. You will find that she may accept a little more help.

Getting the right kind of help can be a frustrating and time-consuming business. Be persistent and do not be put off by unhelpful people. Before you see someone, write down a list of exactly what you want to know from them and also a list of the main problems that you think they may be able to help with. Don't just call in on spec but write or phone for an appointment. Never be afraid to ask to see a more senior person if you feel you are not getting the help you need.

If you get stuck, there are four sources of further advice:

- *Citizens' Advice Bureau.* The address can be found in the local library.
- *Community health council.* A 'watchdog' group committed to acting on behalf of the consumers of the health service. There is one in every health district. Ask to speak to the *secretary.* The phone number is in the telephone directory under the name of the local health district, and is also available at the local library.
- *Your local councillor.* He or she can often 'gee up' the local services on your behalf.
- *Your Member of Parliament.* Write to ask for an appointment to see him or her at one of the local 'surgeries', usually held fortnightly or monthly. Obviously you will want to make a personal approach only if you have a serious grievance, but it does no harm to write and tell your MP about glaring gaps in the local services.

Remember that services are very stretched, and you may be turned down simply because others are judged to be more in need. You may also be turned down because an expert decides that a particular service would not be helpful for your relative. You may have to accept 'no' for an answer.

General practitioners

The important reasons why you should seek help from the sufferer's family doctor as early as possible were mentioned in Chapter 2. You may not be able to persuade them to attend the surgery but you can go along yourself and ask the doctor to visit the person at home. A GP cannot diagnose a patient's condition by 'remote control', and you have every right to insist on a visit if you are concerned about the person's mental health.

What are the chances that you will get a helpful response from the doctor? Unfortunately this is a rather unpredictable business. There are some superb family doctors who take a strong interest in their elderly patients. Some of these have special nurses or social workers who assist them with assessments in the patient's home. Some practices run their own relatives' groups or have a regular routine of revisiting those elderly on their list who are at risk. Such splendid GPs are sadly in the minority. It is reckoned that only one in three GPs has any real interest in his elderly patients, and many GPs regard the elderly as not really worth troubling over; they wrongly assume there is not much to be done. As a general rule, practices in the urban inner-city areas are less likely to be 'good practices' than those in suburban, country-town or rural areas. This is only a generalisation, of course; the best GPs I know work right in the heart of the most deprived areas of London. Fortunately, the overall situation is improving, and now GPs can take an extra diploma qualification to signify that they have special skills in caring for the elderly.

What can the GP do? He can *examine the patient's physical health* and perform some routine *investigations* based on a simple blood test. He can *refer the patient for further assessment* and help from one of the specialist hospital services (see below). He can *prescribe medication* for some of the physical, behavioural and psychological problems discussed earlier. He can *call in specialist therapy help* such as a physiotherapist, an occupational therapist or a speech therapist. As the GP has a responsibility to provide medical care for everyone on his list, he should be the first person you alert about the problem.

Medication

Used with care, the right medicines can help with certain problems. Unfortunately, elderly people are often extra sensitive to the effects of drugs and tend to suffer more than younger people from those unwanted effects that are present to some degree in all medicines. The elderly person's metabolism works more slowly and less efficiently than that of a younger adult. Consequently the older person expels drugs from the body less readily, and there is a tendency for drugs to accumulate in the body. This can slowly lead to a 'drugged' zombie-like state of confusion. This is particularly likely to happen with sedatives such as diazepam (Valium), nitrazepam (Mogadon) and lorazepam (Ativan); these drugs should normally be avoided unless their effects can be very carefully monitored.

Agitation, restlessness, insomnia, hallucinations and delusional ideas can all be helped with the right medication, but the doctor may need to adjust the dosage and type of drug on several occasions before the problem is under control. Too little medication may lead a restless, disturbed person to become noisy and even livelier. Too much and she may become drowsy, incontinent, start to fall, slump sideways, stagger, develop a tremor or become stiff-limbed and immobile. The enlivening effect of a small dose is similar to the effect that alcohol has; one or two drinks will make you feel cheerful and sociable, one or two 'too many' and you feel drunken and drowsy.

The effects of some medications can be even more peculiar. For example, the 'tranquillisers' chlorpromazine (Largactil), promazine (Sparine) and thioridazine (Melleril) are the most efficacious treatments for severe agitation and yet paradoxically they can cause an urge to move around. The patient feels compelled to get up and walk about and cannot sit still for any length of time. It really does need an expert to get the dose right, so don't alter the medication yourself without asking the doctor.

Patients sometimes *refuse* medication or carry a tablet around in the mouth until they can spit it out. This is usually because they are suspicious of the effects of the drug. Giving a drink with the tablet may help. Some patients will accept a liquid syrup medication rather than a tablet, and this is worth trying too. Do not trust the elderly person to take medication without supervision. Hide the bottles in a safe place, preferably a locked cabinet.

There are no miracle cures for dementia

You may read occasionally of a new 'wonder drug' to 'improve the brain circulation' or 'improve the brain's metabolism'. The drug manufacturers have brought out one new drug after another in the last ten years, none of which appears to have any beneficial effect on dementia and which sometimes have the adverse effect of increasing confusion. Research is not yet sufficiently advanced for us to manufacture drugs based on sound scientific principles. All we can do at present is treat some of the symptoms. Fashionable drugs which I do not find effective include Praxilene, Hydergine and Cyclospasmol.

The specialist hospital services

The family doctor can refer a patient suspected of having dementia to a specialist for a second opinion, for a further assessment and for advice on management. There are three types of specialist available: neurologist, geriatrician and psychiatrist/psychogeriatrician.

Neurologist

A neurologist is a specialist in disorders of the brain and nervous system. He is often based at a teaching hospital or specialist neurological centre and has access to advanced technological investigations such as brain scans. You can be sure your relative will get a thorough top-to-toe examination and the right investigations to find treatable causes. Unfortunately, neurologists do not generally interest themselves in providing a continuing service for treatment of symptoms or for the support of the family, and they do not provide hospital beds for long-term care. Neurologists are usually highly gifted doctors; some of the brightest brains in medicine specialise in neurology, and it is sad therefore that so few of them are interested in research or management of one of the commonest neurological illnesses. In a sense they seem to take an interest in the 'technicalities' of neurological disorders, particularly if the case is an unusual one, but no more. Consequently you will usually be offered one or several appointments and investigations but little else.

Geriatrician

A geriatrician is a specialist in the disorders of old age. Geriatricians are essentially physicians dealing with physical illness; nevertheless the majority of geriatricians understand the problems of dementia and in some areas provide the main service. If a person is physically disabled, chairbound or bed-bound by dementia or by a combination of physical and mental disorders, she usually enters a geriatric medical ward for treatment rather than a psychiatric ward. On the other hand a mobile, ambulant patient with dementia who is physically fit is regarded as the responsibility of the psychiatrist or psychogeriatrician. This odd division between the responsibilities of the geriatric and psychiatric services sometimes makes it difficult for the GP to decide who is the best person to refer the patient to, and can lead to delays in getting the right help if the specialist services do not work closely together. Geriatricians usually have facilities for long-term care of physically disabled elderly who need hospital nursing care, but do not usually provide long-term care for the more active, behaviourally disturbed dementia sufferers. This is because geriatric medical ward nurses do not have full psychiatric training but are more 'geared' to the needs of the physically very frail.

Psychiatrist/psychogeriatrician

A psychiatrist is a specialist in mental illnesses. A psychiatrist with a responsibility for providing a service to the elderly may also be called a psychogeriatrician. Psychogeriatricians did not exist until about fifteen years ago, when a small group of psychiatrists began to interest themselves in the growing problems of the elderly with dementia. It is government policy to appoint at least one specialist psychogeriatrician in each health district, and at the time of writing about two-thirds of all districts have their specialists in post. Creating consultant posts in a new speciality is all very well if there are plenty of enthusiastic, well-trained doctors to fill them. Sadly, some of the applicants for psychogeriatric posts have failed to get posts elsewhere and have opted for psychogeriatrics as an easier speciality to enter. A failed general psychiatrist usually ends up as a bad psychogeriatrician. Consequently the quality of the psychogeriatrician can vary enormously from one district to another. Your family doctor will know whether you are likely to get constructive help from your local psychogeriatric service.

What does a psychogeriatrician do? The first important aspect of his work is *assessment*. This means not just taking a full medical history, making an examination and discovering when the illness began and how it developed. It also involves finding out how well the patient functions now in the home setting, what the financial circumstances are, what support the family and neighbours are giving, whether social services are involved and so on. Many consultants believe an initial assessment is best done in the patient's home and see all referrals first in this setting so that they can pick up clues from the conditions at home as to the level of deterioration. Other consultants prefer to see the patient and family together in a day hospital, where a thorough examination can be done, investigations can be performed and a range of professional therapists can assess the patient more fully. The way the consultant chooses to work will depend on which area he covers (in a vast rural area it is more difficult to offer instant assessment at home), the supporting staff he has to help him and his facilities. The author, for example, has no day hospital and few in-patient beds but does have an excellent team of professional therapists and nurses who are able to offer early assessment at home.

Once the assessment is complete, the consultant and his team will plan a care 'package' or treatment plan. This might include advice on medication, a request to the local day centre for two days' attendance to give family relief, regular follow-up visits by a community psychiatric nurse to help the carer deal more effectively with a difficult behaviour problem and so on. Few patients need urgent admission to hospital, but if the patient appears to have an illness that needs hospital treatment, or if the medical problems are very complex and need more intensive assessment, a short hospital admission may be recommended.

Many relatives and, of course, patients themselves are concerned that the specialist may recommend that the patient be admitted to a mental hospital for long-stay care and will not offer anything else. This is not the case. The consultant's main aim is to help you and the patient cope as best as possible without removing the patient. Indeed, the consultant is rarely able to offer instant, permanent admission for long-stay care even if that is what you want. It is not just that such places are in short supply; the consultant also has to consider the needs and wishes of the patient as well as those of the family, and often has to ration his resources to make sure that those in most urgent need get priority.

Nursing and other health services

Community psychiatric nurses

'CPNs' have emerged in recent years as the major providers of home treatment and support of mentally ill patients living in the general community. They are all fully trained psychiatric nurses, often with general medical nurse training as well, working at 'ward sister' level and above. Their 'ward' is the local community instead of a hospital ward. Some work in the psychogeriatrician's team, based in the hospital. Others are based in health centres and take referrals from GPs and social workers as well as from the consultant. The role of the CPN is a difficult one. She often carries enormous responsibility for the support and supervision of patients at home and has to liaise effectively with social services, the GP and the hospital services. If these back-up services are inadequate, she will not be able to help very much. CPNs do not normally carry out physical nursing tasks such as changing dressings, bathing and feeding, but do give injections of some medications. Physical care tasks usually fall to district nurses.

District nurses

Also called community nurses, district nurses are the main providers of physical care and treatment in the home. They are usually attached to general practices or work from health centres or community clinics. In many areas district nurses or their auxiliary nurse helpers will get patients up and dressed in the mornings, regularly bath the patient, supervise medication, change dressings and provide a 'tucking in' service at night. District nurses can provide advice on incontinence, bowel problems and diet. They usually carry an enormous work-load, and in some areas there are too few of them to supervise daily medication or provide a night nursing service. This is a pity since a good district nursing service can be of immeasurable practical help. District nurses frequently deal with confused old people and yet have little training in psychiatric nursing. Some are not confident to handle seriously disturbed patients and do not understand dementia or severe depression, and this can be a drawback to helping a family with a dementia sufferer.

The district nurse can arrange the loan of bottles and commodes and organise supplies of incontinence pads and aids. She can also arrange for the incontinence laundry service to call. To contact a district nurse, ask at your GP's surgery.

Incontinence laundry services

Many districts now offer a service to collect and launder soiled bed linen. They usually pick up and deliver on a weekly basis, which means you have to have lots of linen! Someone has to prepare the linen ready for collection and receive the bag of fresh laundry, so this service doesn't work well for a dementia sufferer living alone who will not be able to organise it. Ask the district nurse for details.

Health visitors

Health visitors are qualified nurses whose main task is to give advice and education to families with young babies. Their role is educational and preventive. A few also work with the elderly, but the majority do not. At a time when the birth rate is falling but the proportion of severely disabled elderly is rising, I think it is about time we rethought the responsibilities of health visitors.

Occupational therapists

'OTs' are neither nurses nor doctors but are highly trained specialist therapists. Their main task is sorting out the problems that a person has in managing the tasks of daily life. These may be physical tasks, like getting out of bed and dressing, or mental tasks such as making a shopping list and preparing food. Although most OTs work in hospital teams alongside doctors and nurses, an increasing number are primarily community based and offer a domiciliary service, working with a psychiatric community team. They assess how well a person can perform the activities of daily living, their mental functioning and their need for practical aids. A skilled OT who is experienced in psychogeriatric work will also take on a supportive and counselling role to the patient and her family. OTs are scarce on the ground unfortunately, so not every service has one.

Psychologists

These should not be confused with psychiatrists. Psychiatrists are medical doctors, whereas clinical psychologists are not doctors but have a specialist degree and postgraduate qualification in the function of the human mind. They have special skills in assessing the various functions of the brain. Most spend much of their time in counselling and devising courses of treatment based on the principles of learning. For example, when a patient has become housebound due to having lost confidence after an illness a psychologist may be called in to help 'teach' that person how to get out and about again. Psychologists are extremely useful when working within a multi-disciplinary team. There are as yet only a handful of psychologists specifically devoted to working in the community with elderly patients, but the numbers are growing.

Services provided by the local authority

The social services department of your local authority can be located by enquiring at the town hall or by looking it up in the telephone directory. The services are usually divided into areas and are based at offices in the locality they serve.

Home helps

This service is the backbone of community support for the elderly and for those with mild and moderate degrees of dementia living alone. Home helps are often the main providers of the practical care that allows elderly people to remain in their own homes. The quality and quantity of the service vary from area to area. On the whole, home helps do far, far more than just the cleaning and shopping jobs usually expected of them; they often give personal care help to their clients and become friends as well.

Some authorities, recognising the need for more intensive, personal help for some individuals, have set up special teams of home helps who carry out work half-way between that of an ordinary home help and that of an auxiliary nurse. They may do household chores, bathing, dressing, washing clothes, cooking meals and so on. These special home helps are variously called 'home care aides', 'domiciliary care assistants' and 'care attendants'. Where they exist they are a magnificent addition to the service.

Problems can crop up in connection with home helps when the client has dementia. The client may forget who the help is and refuse to let her in. The helper may be wrongly accused of stealing the client's money or treasured possessions. The client may not wish to pay the modest fee for the service. The home may become so dirty and unkempt that the help finds it too unpleasant to continue her visits. These problems can be overcome, but obviously it is essential to have a trustworthy and tactful home help with plenty of common sense and tolerance.

To contact the home help service, ask for the home care organiser for your local area at the social services office.

Meals-on-wheels

Social services departments either provide a meals delivery service or subcontract the service to a local voluntary agency, such as the WRVS or Age Concern. The aim is to deliver a nutritious midday meal on several or all days of the week to those who are unable to prepare their own food. This sounds fine and in practice it works well for mentally alert, disabled elderly people. The meals are meant to be hot but are often delivered lukewarm or cold in an aluminium carton, which then has to be heated in the oven at home. The person delivering the meal does not supervise the consuming of it. For the person with dementia who may need reminding to eat, the meals-on-wheels service may be useless unless there is someone available to warm the food, prepare it on the plate ready for eating and then supervise the meal. The quality of the meals is also variable; they tend to look like unappetising school dinners and do not on the whole cater for individual tastes or ethnic minorities. An exception to this is the kosher meals-on-wheels service for the orthodox Jewish population in some parts of the country.

Social workers

Social workers are highly trained professional staff employed by social services departments. They have an extensive training for a wide range of tasks. They are concerned with assessment of an individual's need for provision of appropriate services, and have skills in counselling and helping people tackle crises and periods of change in their lives. Social workers can support families with problems, are experts at assessing 'risk' and should know when to begin to talk with an elderly person about the need for residential care. On a practical front they are the gateway for admission to a local authority old people's home since it is they who make the application and assessment.

Like doctors, however, social workers have not on the whole been trained to recognise the potential for work with the elderly. Working with the elderly tends to have low status and is often delegated to untrained 'social work assistants' or 'social welfare officers', who have little or no understanding of the problems of a patient with dementia. The consequence is that a familiar train of events can be triggered. It goes like this: a social worker visits someone to assess the need for home help, meals-on-wheels, etc. The elderly woman with dementia says she doesn't want any services. The social worker accepts the refusal at its face value, unaware that the patient is unable to make a rational judgement about her need for assistance. The social worker then happily closes the case and doesn't call again. Or perhaps the patient has been referred for consideration for an old people's home. Again the patient is interviewed, adamantly rejects the suggestion in spite of the clear evidence of failure to cope, the social worker accepts this and again closes the case.

The situation is improving. Many boroughs now have specialist teams of social workers for the elderly. Most psychogeriatricians have social workers attached to their teams who liaise with the community-based area social workers. A social worker who is prepared to work with an elderly person and the family can be of enormous help in ensuring that a skilled assessment is carried out and a properly planned support service instituted.

Day care

Most day centres for the elderly are run by local authorities, although some are run by voluntary agencies. A few boroughs have day centres specially for the elderly with dementia. The function of a day centre for this group of people is to provide a stimulating, enjoyable environment in which the elderly person can be encouraged to maintain practical and social skills and hence help prevent social deterioration. If your relative lives alone it can be reassuring to know that two or three days a week she is attending a centre where she will get a properly supervised meal and someone keeping an eye on her. For those with a relative living with them, a break from the strain, a little time to themselves, may be invaluable.

As usual, however, there are drawbacks. The more the demented person and her caring family need day care to relieve the strain, the less likely they are to be offered it. Day centres do not feel they can cope with seriously disturbed dementia sufferers. Even day centres for the confused do not deal very effectively with incontinence. Staff do not like 'wanderers' or those who show aggressive outbursts of temper, who are noisy or who are both physically and mentally disabled. Tolerance of these problems depends very much on the qualities of the manager. If you possibly can, it is helpful to meet the manager beforehand and describe any problems, so that she can be forewarned.

Day care can rarely be organised instantly because of the wait for a 'transport' place. If you can organise your own transport, a place may be offered more quickly.

Relatives are not always eager to take advantage of day care. You may find it hard to hand over your loved one for the day because of your feelings of embarrassment about her behaviour and what other people might think. It is sometimes difficult letting go of the responsibility to someone else; this is why it is important to meet the manager and talk over the problems first. Remember too that it will take the elderly person some time to get used to the centre and longer still for her to become friendly with other attenders, so do not be surprised if she appears distressed after the first few visits. Persevere, and she will usually settle.

Problems of transport, difficulties in getting the person

ready for the ambulance in time, the reluctance of elderly
people to attend, the eccentric hours (normally 10.00 a.m. to
3.00 p.m.: not day care but midday care) – all these prevent
day care from being a more useful facility for working
carers.

People with severe dementia who are living alone cannot
usually be sustained effectively just by a day care centre.
They fail to remember the minibus is coming, or may go for a
whole weekend without eating and drinking. During
unsupervised nights the individual remains at risk.

Day hospitals

Day hospitals and day centres are often difficult to
distinguish from one another. Day hospitals for the elderly
mentally ill are run by the local health service, not the local
authority or voluntary agency (as in the case of day centres).
Many psychogeriatricians use their day hospitals as their
main assessment centres. The social aspects of day care for
long-term support and relief are provided by some day
hospitals, usually because day care centres will not take
more severely confused patients. But a day hospital cannot
provide both an effective assessment service for new
patients and social care as well. Patients attending for long-
term support are often offered little in the way of
stimulation and activities. Day hospitals share the same
transport and 'hours' problems as day centres.

Night sitters

Some local authority social services departments can provide
a night sitter who will stay awake in the home one or two
nights a week to enable a caring relative to get a full night's
sleep. Sleep deprivation is one of the most wearing, stressful
effects of caring for a dementia sufferer. Even on the nights
when the patient appears to be sleeping soundly it is
difficult for the carer to relax, knowing that at any minute
the sick person may be up and about in a confused state.
Departments that do have a night-sitter service are not

normally very forthcoming about advertising the fact; it is an expensive service to provide, and they use it sparingly. It is also rarely available for more than one or two nights a week or up to three or four nights in a crisis. Clients are usually charged a small fee that is only a fraction of the real cost.

As you can imagine, it is difficult to attract the right kind of staff to do this demanding work. Moreover, the client's family may find it difficult to tolerate a stranger in the house at night while they are asleep. The fear of embarrassment or of too much burden being laid on the shoulders of someone outside the family circle is a difficult feeling to allay. Night sitters can nevertheless be a godsend, and close friendships sometimes grow up between regular sitters and their 'families'. Sadly, only half of our social services departments provide such a service at present.

Holidays

You may have wondered if a holiday away from home would brighten up the elderly person. Would a change of scenery be cheering and stimulating? Holidays away from home are unfortunately usually difficult, sometimes disastrous. The unfamiliarity of a hotel room or self-catering flat often worsens confusion, especially at night. Travelling can be a heavy strain on the carer; at the end of the journey you may feel you know the way to every public convenience *en route*. Travelling by air can cause serious problems for patients with multi-infarct dementia, who may develop transient signs of stroke or worsening confusion during the flight, arriving in a confused, bewildered state. If you are travelling to relatives who understand the problems and are going to share the burden for a while, the difficulties may still be worth putting up with.

You, the carer, however, definitely need a good annual or six-monthly break. If you have no relatives who are prepared to take over the burden for a week or two, approach your local social services department or your doctor about the possibility of a short break. If the dementia sufferer is mobile, mildly confused and continent, the local authority will usually be able to offer a short-term place in a local authority old people's home. If the individual is more seriously confused or has disturbed behaviour or heavy incontinence, short-term care will more appropriately be provided in hospital by the psychogeriatrician. Almost all psychogeriatricians and geriatricians offer 'holiday relief', recognising that if you were not able to care for them for the other fifty weeks of a year the patient would almost certainly be occupying one of their long-stay beds.

Points to remember:

(1) Start asking in January and get a definite booking for a summer holiday.

(2) Go away somewhere when your relative goes for the break. It's no rest for you to keep rushing up to the home or hospital to make sure the patient's 'settled'.

(3) A person with dementia *will* get more confused away from home and possibly on returning home. This is a temporary thing but to be expected.

(4) *Label* your relative's clothes, spectacles, hearing-aid, handbag and so on with her name. If you can, ask your dentist to label any dentures with a distinctive mark.

(5) Take all medication in clearly labelled bottles and make sure someone at the home or hospital understands how to give it.

(6) The staff haven't got eyes in the back of their heads and they have many more people to care for than just the one for whom you care. So if your relative wanders off, perhaps looking for home, try not to be cross with the staff, who will already be feeling anxious and guilty about it.

(7) There will usually be a charge for a stay in an old people's home, assessed on the elderly person's income and assets.

Help from voluntary organisations

Some of the most original ideas for providing help for dementia sufferers and their carers have come from voluntary bodies. The main national ones are listed in the Appendix, but all over the country groups have sprung up to serve local needs. Voluntary organisations providing services specifically for confused elderly people are usually started by an enterprising relative, by a local church group or as an offshoot of one of the national organisations. Many groups run day centres, 'drop-in' centres, or 'lunch clubs'. Others provide voluntary visitors and sitters to allow a few hours' relief during the day. One of the best-known 'sitting' schemes in Britain is the Crossroads Care Attendant Scheme, named after *Crossroads*, the ATV serial. ATV helped finance the first pilot scheme in Rugby. Crossroads groups provide sitters and carers who will perform personal tasks for handicapped people of all ages living in the community. Not all Crossroads groups are willing to take on the task of caring for a dementia sufferer, but some will.

The range of services provided by voluntary organisations varies so widely across the country that you have to enquire locally to find out what is available in your area. Contact the local volunteer bureau, or the voluntary services officer at the social services office.

Mutual support groups

Such groups for relatives are run by many branches of Age Concern, the Alzheimer's Disease Society and other organisations (see Chapter 4, pages 63–5).

Buying in private help

This is an expensive option for most families but you may be able to find a local person who will sit for a few hours with your relative for a reasonable hourly payment. You have to be certain the person can cope with the problems and understands the patient's needs. You might also consider buying in help with cleaning and shopping, simply to relieve you of part of the weekly chores. If you can afford it, private nursing agencies can provide a night nurse to sit with the patient a few nights of the week; look them up under 'nurses' in your local Yellow Pages. In London and some other parts of Britain there are reliable private night-caring services that specialise in providing services to families with an elderly person.

Fostering schemes

You will have heard of fostering children with families. There are also a few areas in which an elderly person can be taken to stay for a short time in someone else's home. These 'boarding-out' schemes are not very useful for someone with severe dementia but can work for the mildly confused if the fostering family is well prepared and supported. Ask your local social services department if there is a scheme of this kind locally. An elderly person often finds it easier to settle in a familiar home-like environment than in an institution.

There has recently been a proliferation of innovative services that can help to lighten the burden of care. There will be help somewhere in your local area if you persist in your search, so it really is worth digging around to find out who can best help with your particular problem.

6

Residential Care

In Britain elderly people generally prefer to live alone rather than share a home with their children, brothers or sisters. They like to see their families frequently and like to feel that they can call on them when needed, but few desire to move in with them. They want to preserve their independence for as long as possible. Moreover, children rarely want to have their parents in the same house day after day. However close you may feel to your parents, there are differences between generations that frequently lead to a tense and unhappy atmosphere when two or more generations of one family live together. One-third of the elderly population live alone in their own homes, and only 6 per cent live with their children.

An elderly person with dementia who is used to living alone is consequently usually reluctant to move. However, it often eventually becomes clear to everyone around that the person cannot continue to live alone. If an individual is eating insufficient food and therefore losing weight, cannot use a fire, a kettle or stove safely and is becoming a serious fire hazard, the risk of leaving the person on their own is usually considered by relatives and professionals to be too great. Persistent incontinence and soiling or frequent wandering out at night are also very difficult to manage when someone lives alone. If the individual refuses to have help from the home care services, a crisis may be reached quickly; there comes a time when all agree that the sufferer needs to live in an environment where she can be supervised for twenty-four hours a day.

'Should she come to live with us?'

The decision as to whether or not you can care for an elderly person in your own home is a major one, which changes the lives of both the family and the elderly person. It is not something to be undertaken without a great deal of thought. If the elderly person is your relative, how does your husband or wife feel? What was their relationship like before he or she developed dementia? However close and devoted you feel to your mother or father, your spouse's feelings should be considered carefully. However strong your marriage, the presence of a dependent confused person poses an enormous strain, particularly on the wife, who generally undertakes most of the personal care tasks. This can lead to quarrels between the caring couple. If there is resentment and reluctance by either partner towards having a 'cuckoo' in the nest the new arrangement will probably affect the marriage adversely.

Remember what the practical caring tasks will be and the impact on the daily routine. The couple may not be able to go out together in the evenings without finding a sitter. Nights may be disturbed; sensible conversation may be possible only when the two are alone together. They may never be able to watch the TV in peace without being interrupted by someone pacing around. Often there is simply not enough room; the elderly person needs a room of her own.

Consider carefully the effect on any children in the house. Small children and babies are generally unperturbed by confused people. They take their lead from adults. If adults have tolerant and kindly attitudes towards the sufferer, so will they. Nor are young children generally upset or adversely affected in their emotional development by the presence of a disturbed person, although it is important for them to be told why Granny is forgetful or gets funny ideas. Even children at toddler age can understand that an illness affects the way people behave and that the sufferer needs caring for. But as they become young teenagers they will become more self-conscious about the way their family appears to their friends and they may find the confused person embarrassing and upsetting. It is important not to keep the children in the dark about the real problems, tempting though it is not to worry them, particularly when they are working for examinations. They can and should share the responsibilities of caring.

'Do I like this person?'

All of us generally get along with one parent better than with another. You can love someone, be deeply attached to them and worry about them and yet not be able to spend more than twenty-four hours together because of a lifelong dislike of their habits, attitudes and opinions. This is especially true for those who never got on well with their parents when they were children. These interpersonal tensions do not go away when the elderly person comes to live in the same house; usually the relationship gets worse.

'Why don't we sell our house and hers and get a bigger one for both of us?'

One temptation for a couple with a growing family and who have a confused parent who owns a home is to sell both homes and have the parent to live with them in a jointly financed larger home. This arrangement can work well where a mentally alert elderly person can have her own 'granny flat' and live independently. But a confused person has to live as part of the family because she will be unable to use separate 'quarters' or rooms of her own.

If a time then comes when the family feels that the strain is too much and the dementia sufferer needs residential care, all the elderly person's capital to pay for this care may be tied up in the new house. Money is therefore not available for meeting the cost of a good private home. The caring children may find it difficult to arrange residential care through the statutory services, and, furthermore, the local authority has the power to place a charge over the elderly person's assets to pay for the care. This may mean that the family cannot move house without first paying back the local authority. This financial trap often leads desperate families to go on caring long after they are able to do it effectively. In practice many local authorities do not, at present, place a charge over jointly owned assets in order to pay for care. Some do, however, and it is always possible that in the future local authorities will be left no option as to whether to be 'generous' or not in this matter.

Don't have your relative to live with you simply for the sake of duty

Consider your own strengths and talents but your weaknesses too, your family life, your health, your future plans, your finances and most importantly your love and liking for this person in the past.

Choosing residential care

Dementia sufferers do not improve with time. They normally become more dependent on others for personal care and gradually become less like the people they once were, losing the ability to maintain a relationship with those who care for them. There may come a time when the most important thing is a comfortable physical environment and skilled nursing care. At this point they may be unable to recognise who is doing the caring. The carers must ask themselves whether they can really provide this kind of care even with help. Families are often worried about the alternatives to continuing to care at home. By the time the decision is made to find a residential place, the person is often too disabled to be managed satisfactorily in an old people's home. The only course of action may be nursing care, and this may be available locally only in a psychiatric ward in a mental hospital or in a geriatric medical ward of an old general hospital. The stigma of placing a relative in an 'asylum' or 'workhouse' or 'loony bin' often gives relatives a totally wrong idea of what these places are like now. Those large Victorian institutions are not all perfect by any means but the vast majority of mental hospitals have set aside special wards for the elderly mentally ill where the patients will not be mixed together with patients with other mental disorders. Many hospitals have upgraded and improved the wards. If this is your worry, ask to visit the hospital in question. The social worker or consultant involved is usually happy to arrange this.

In practice, the decision is often taken out of the family's hands, for example as a result of a crisis such as the ill-health of the patient or the carer. It is usually the professional workers involved in the case who will ultimately make the decision by offering a continuing care place. Whoever makes the decision, it is a painful and distressing one for the carer. The decision is especially painful for a caring spouse, who in effect is separating permanently from the person they have been married to perhaps for half a century. The spouse feels that they have let the patient down, that they should have been able to cope, that they are guilty of weakness and have abandoned the loved person. Simply removing a familiar face from the house may leave the remaining spouse feeling isolated, lonely and fearful of the future. Relief from the burden of caring is often just as difficult to cope with as the burden itself.

The feelings of grief and guilt at placing an elderly relative in care are usually present to some degree in caring children but normally to a lesser extent than in a spouse. The overriding feeling of relief from the trap of day-to-day care usually far outweighs the negative feelings. The sense of freedom that relatives feel when a confused person finally accepts residential care is often remarkable: no more anxious phone calls from neighbours in the middle of the night, no more worrying about fire risks and accidents, no more perpetual cleaning up the home, and so on.

Persuading the person to move

As has been mentioned, most elderly people do not want to leave the familiarity of their own home, give up their independence and enter a nursing home or hospital. The elderly of today remember only too well the horror of the workhouse and the inflexible charity handed out by the public institutions. 'You're trying to put me away' is a common fear. If this is your problem at the moment, the first question you should ask yourself is *why* you want her to move into a home. Is it because of the strain on you? If it is, try to think whether or not she could survive on her own without your assistance if she had more statutory services (Chapter 5) or whether you can cope a little longer. If she cannot manage alone and refuses to have any other help than yourself, then you are justified in deciding to place her in care if the strain is becoming more than you can tolerate.

On the other hand, if someone else bears the main responsibility for caring, the decision should rest with that other person. I often meet families in which one adult child who is carrying the day-to-day responsibility feels that she is at breaking-point and cannot continue; but the other children, whose contribution is much less onerous, do not approve of the decision to place the elderly person in residential care, although they are happy to allow their brother or sister to carry on the struggle. The person who provides the roof over the patient's head and does the physical caring is the one who should make the decision.

Talk it over with the elderly person as soon as possible. In the early and 'middling' stages of dementia, sufferers are very sensitive to discussions within the family. They soon pick up that their future is being discussed, that decisions about sending them into residential care are about to be made. The anxiety and resentment this generates can be very hard for carers to tolerate. But however painful this is for the carer, the person must be told face to face of any plans. Do not leave it to a social worker or other professional, because the sufferer often gets the idea that her own family do not support the idea. This can lead to protracted problems, with the elderly relative becoming puzzled and resentful as the family members fail to involve themselves in the arguments.

Be honest with the person about the reasons for residential care. 'It's for your own good' is not a very helpful statement. Rather, use an example of the worry you have had, e.g. 'The day I found you burning the saucepans reminded me that you don't always remember to eat your meals. You've lost weight now, and your health is deteriorating. I want to see you cared for.' Or if the person concerned is living with you in your own home, be honest about the effect on you, your health and your family and don't imply that the decision is being made solely for the patient's sake.

Disadvantages

Residential care has some disadvantages for those used to living alone. Giving up one's own home is often a devastating experience for a mentally impaired elderly person. No one who has witnessed the perplexed grief and despair of a disorientated elderly patient in the days immediately after admission can doubt the adverse impact of an involuntary admission to a residential home. Constant perplexed searching for familiar people, wandering back to the old neighbourhood, increased agitation and tearfulness – these are common phenomena associated with institutionalisation.

People who have been independent and inclined to shun the company of others find the 'boarding-school' atmosphere of many old people's homes intolerably crowded and wearisomely noisy. There is often little privacy, and the only way to keep one's distance is to withdraw into a private world where the individual communicates as little as possible with other residents and staff. Residents who are poor mixers sometimes get labelled as 'stubborn', 'difficult' or 'isolated'. Communal life is difficult enough for many people to tolerate when they are young and fit; Butlin's and Club Méditerranée holidays are not everyone's ideal. Imagine what an old people's home can be like after getting comfortably used to ten or twenty years of living alone.

It is also important to consider whether the person being admitted to care is really going to be safer from accidents and provided with better physical care. There is evidence that those who are prone to fall, for example, are just as much at risk in an institution as at home. You may be reassured that at least your relative will not lie on the floor all night in pain with no one to pick her up. This is a comparatively rare occurrence, however, and does not in itself generally warrant an admission for care. Furthermore, there is some evidence that the move itself may predispose elderly people to developing illnesses and increased confusion.

It is extremely difficult to stand by and watch a loved relative living in increasing squalor, forgetting to wash and change, eating God-knows-what and clearly managing to survive only by the presence of the home care services and luck. The natural instinct is to want the person cared for by professional, understanding people in a 'nice home'. But it is often more courageous and understanding to allow an elderly relative the dignity and freedom of remaining in their own home to the last. If you are making this decision, consider the sort of person the individual is. What would this individual's view be if she were able to make a rational judgement about her own future?

Options for residential care

Local Authority Old People's Homes ('Part III' homes)

Local authority residential homes provide for elderly people in numbers ranging from twenty to two hundred. Most have fifty to sixty places in one home. These homes were established as a result of the 1948 National Assistance Act. They may be called 'Part III' homes because they are mentioned in Part III of the 1948 Act. You may hear social workers and doctors talking about 'going into Part III', and this is jargon for admission to a local authority home. Nye Bevan, the Labour politician, was one of the prime movers of the idea to replace the ghastly, huge, Poor Law institutions. His dream for the elderly was to create decent hostel-like accommodation where those in need of help could live a sheltered but communal life, served by a small staff of domestic workers providing meals and the occasional bit of help. The idea was to have 'hotels' for alert but frail old people. The homes grew in number over the next thirty years, more or less keeping pace with the growth of the elderly population, although there has been a slowing down recently because of general restrictions on the growth of local authority services. This has coincided with a strong increase in the numbers of elderly; so in recent years a 'gap' has opened up between the need and the availability of 'Part III' beds.

These homes never quite worked out in practice as Bevan intended. Elderly people became financially more secure with the rise in old age pensions. They wanted to preserve their independence in their own homes and, as pensions increased, they could usually afford to do so. Fit people didn't need these 'hotel' services. At the same time, the growing numbers of very frail and mentally impaired elderly *did* need residential care, so it was they who ended up filling these homes.

We now have a very odd situation in Britain. Two-thirds of the residents of 'Part III' homes are suffering from dementia, and yet the local authorities usually provide very little nursing care in these homes. 'Part III' homes are usually poorly staffed, may have no trained nurses at all and sometimes only superficial links with the medical services. They nevertheless provide the majority of the residential places available in this country for the care of elderly people with dementia.

Getting a place. The 'gatekeeper' to a 'Part III' home is a social worker. The usual procedure is for a social worker to make a formal application to the residential services division of social services on behalf of the elderly person. In many boroughs there is an expert panel of senior social workers and managers, who meet every week or two to consider applications in depth. The social worker on the case will present the social, psychological and medical facts available about the person to the panel, who will then decide first if the client is suitable for a place in 'Part III' and, if so, how quickly admission should be arranged. In theory this is fine, but vacancies arise randomly in the local homes, and inevitably the panel finds itself slotting people into vacancies as and when they arise rather than starting with a person's needs and finding an appropriate place at the appropriate time. Thus a place may be available quickly but in a home some miles away, while a place in a nearby home may not arise for months.

A major part of a social worker's job is to assess the need and to help towards making an appropriate decision at the right time. The social worker will be familiar with the local council's policy on the admission of confused residents, whether or not the homes will accept people with incontinence or behaviour disorders and so on. Although the criteria vary widely from one council to another, the more seriously confused, those who wander and those who are behaviourly disturbed are generally not welcomed. Incontinence has to be occasional rather than persistent. Patients must be able to walk unaided unless they are alert and able to manage their own walking-frames or wheelchairs. These entrance criteria are understandable if you remember that the staff are usually untrained to deal with mentally ill people and are essentially employed as domestics. The senior care staff of these homes do have some professional training in caring for the elderly but again, usually, no specific training in dementia and other mental problems of old age.

The upshot of these criteria is that the more your relative needs residential care, the less likely she is to be eligible for 'Part III'. The local authorities say that it is 'the National Health's job', i.e. the hospitals' responsibility, to provide care for the severely demented person. In reality there are far too few appropriate hospital places for these patients; a person may fall into the trap in the middle: 'too good for hospital, too bad for Part III'.

If you are offered a 'Part III' place, don't expect necessarily to have a choice of home. You may have looked around one near by and liked it. But remember that if you wait for a place in one particular home, you may have to wait months. You will probably have little choice but to accept the first vacancy offered if speed of placement is important. If you don't mind waiting, you can afford to press the social worker for the home of your choice.

The physical environment of 'Part IIIs' varies considerably from one authority to another and even within one area. Some are large converted Victorian houses; others are purpose-built modern homes. The following remarks about choosing a private home should be borne in mind when you first look at a local authority home.

Remember that your elderly relative will be paying the local authority for residential care. It is not charity. Even though the contribution may be small if the person has no personal savings, the elderly person has very likely been paying rates to that council for a long time and has therefore been contributing indirectly to the old people's homes. So don't be afraid to ask for what you want, be prepared to criticise if you don't like what you see and don't be afraid to complain to the head of the home or to more senior managers in the residential services department in the local town hall offices if necessary.

The cost of a place in 'Part III' to the resident is a complicated business, but the charges are worked out on the principle that a resident should pay what he or she can afford as a contribution to board, lodging and care, up to the full cost of a place. There are national guidelines for charging, which you can read in DHSS booklet *Residential Homes: Charging and Assessment*. This is available from social security offices and social services departments. However these guidelines are interpreted with varying degrees of latitude by local authorities.

A person who has national insurance pension income only, but no property or savings, will pay most of their pension towards the cost of their keep and will be left with a small sum for personal spending on toiletries, cigarettes and so on. Some small amount of personal savings and a small proportion of private income are exempt. On the other hand, a person who owns property or other substantial assets will be assessed for a much larger contribution to weekly charges, and most residents are obliged to sell their former home in order to meet the charges. The council cannot compel a person to sell their former house, but in those circumstances on the death of the individual a claim may be made against the estate. A local authority may, as mentioned before, exercise discretion with regard to an elderly person's property where it is also occupied by children as a family home or where property is jointly owned by the elderly person and a spouse or other relatives. It is therefore important to check exactly what the charges will be. If there are any problems, discuss them with the finance officer in the social services department.

Voluntary and charitable homes

There are now a large number of religious organisations and charities that build and run old people's homes. Conditions for admission to many of these homes are that the resident is a member of the church group or satisfies the criteria laid down by the charitable foundation for recipients of the charity. For example, Methodist Homes for the Aged are specially for elderly Methodists; the Licensed Victuallers' Association runs homes for retired publicans. There are homes for retired sailors, nurses, firemen, policemen, actors and so on. If your relative belonged to a specific profession, group or trade union it is worth making enquiries about the availability of a special home. Many voluntary homes do not have exclusive criteria and are prepared to consider any elderly person in need. However, few of these homes are willing to take individuals with severe dementia and it is worth checking this point when making enquiries. Charges in voluntary and charitable homes are usually assessed by a 'means test' similar to that used for local authority homes.

Private rest homes

If the elderly person owns their own property or has a substantial private income, or has children or other relatives prepared to contribute financially, a private home is worth thinking about. The best homes are private, although the worst homes are private too. There is enormous variation in the quality of care, and this is not just a reflection of how much is being charged. You do not necessarily get better care by paying more. So how do you find a private home to suit your relative?

First you will need a list of 'registered homes' from the local authority. You can get such a list from the town hall or from a social worker. After your surprise at the sheer number of homes to consider, ring them up in turn, explain fully what your elderly relative's problems are and how much help they need and get an idea as to whether or not the home is prepared to consider a confused elderly person. If it sounds promising, make an appointment to visit and have a talk with the matron or manager in day-to-day charge of the home.

Looking round the home. When you visit, make sure you get an opportunity to have a good look round. Consider the following points:

- *Do residents have their own room and washing facilities?* If not, how is sharing organised? Can residents bring their own furniture and personal possessions? Is there room for storing clothes and other items? Is there a comfortable chair in the bedroom? Is the floor in the bedroom non-slip? Have existing residents been encouraged to put up photos, pictures and knick-knacks of their own? Is the heating adequate and safe in bedrooms? How many toilets are there for the residents? How many bathrooms? Are there any aids in the WC and bathroom for those with physical handicaps?
- *Are the communal sitting rooms large enough?* Does the seating arrangement look as if it encourages residents to

talk to each other? Was there a conversation going on when you looked in or was it all deathly silence?

- *Is the home clean? Does it smell of urine?* A good home knows how to deal effectively with incontinence and does not smell. The home should look clean and well cared for but not necessarily tidy; a bit of homely chaos sometimes indicates that there is more activity going on.

- *What activities are available?* Was the TV or radio blaring away inappropriately the day you visited? Does anyone come in to organise music programmes, joint activities, group games? What outings are arranged for the residents? How much exercise do the residents get? Are the outings included in the weekly charge, or do they charge extra? Is there anyone employed to organise activities?

- *Do the staff seem friendly and helpful?* Is the manager/matron the sort of person you would trust to be kindly and tolerant? Are all your questions answered openly and honestly? Is there a warm atmosphere in the residents' lounge?

- *What medical help is available to the home?* Is there a regular 'surgery' held by the doctor who visits the home? Can the residents remain registered with their own GP if they wish? Who gives out prescribed medication? Is the home able to provide a chiropody service or physiotherapist when required?

- *What time of day are meals served?* Does the day start at a reasonable hour? Early morning tea at 6.00 a.m. is *not* reasonable unless it's the specific wish of a resident to be up at the crack of dawn. Similarly, a last meal at four o'clock in the afternoon is not common practice outside of institutions. If you can, have a look at the food offered at mealtimes; would *you* want to eat it?

- *Charges.* Make sure you know exactly what is being offered as inclusive with the weekly charges. Laundry bills, outings, special activities and medical bills are all charged extra in some establishments.

- *Visiting: are there restrictions?* There should be no fixed visiting hours, and in general you should be able to visit whenever and in however large a group you wish, babies and children included. (Bear in mind, however, that a crowd is not always very easy for a confused person to cope with.)

- Will the resident be asked to leave if his or her mental or physical condition deteriorates? If so, what arrangements does the home have with the local authority and district hospitals service?

It is worth considering these issues very carefully. I know private rest homes where patients are treated harshly and insensitively. They may look relatively clean and smart but are totally joyless. Others I know look rather more disorganised but are caring and friendly. Take time to make an assessment. If you have any doubts have a friend or relative visit for a second opinion or try elsewhere.

Private Nursing Homes

Private rest homes do not necessarily have nursing staff round the clock and are not expected to provide basic personal care and physical nursing care, although many do. Nursing homes, on the other hand, must be registered with the local district health authority and must provide twenty-four-hour qualified nursing cover. A nursing home can usually provide the same kind of skilled nursing as an ordinary hospital, but there is usually little medical input and few facilities for investigation and active treatment of the kind you would expect in a general hospital. Nursing homes are more expensive than rest homes but they do not necessarily provide more appropriate care for a confused elderly person. They are usually geared to the frail, immobile elderly and have little space for activities and communal living. Some do welcome dementia sufferers, but it is most important to check this out when making your enquiries. You should investigate the facilities at a nursing home with the same care as for rest homes.

The move into residential care

When the decision has been made, tell the elderly person as soon as possible and arrange for her to visit the home to meet the staff and have a look around. You may feel this is a waste of time for someone with a very short memory who may have apparently forgotten all about the visit by the next day, but it is usually worth arranging this introduction, particularly in the company of a trusted relative.

On the day of admission, ensure that a close relative or friend accompanies the elderly person and stays with them for a while. This is especially important if the individual is being transferred direct from a stay in hospital to a permanent home. Imagine the bewilderment of a mentally impaired person who is taken by ambulance to an unfamiliar place and left there with a group of strangers.

Make sure the admission has a trial period of four to six weeks at first and do not make arrangements to sell or give up renting the elderly person's home until you are completely sure the person has settled. Be prepared to change homes if you are not happy with the standard of care provided. The social worker will want to discuss a placement in 'Part III' with relatives and the staff of the home a few weeks after admission so as to review any problems and ensure that the placement is an appropriate one. In the case of a private home a relative ought to do this on behalf of the elderly person.

Visit frequently during the first few days and weeks. The feelings of abandonment and confusion that a dementia sufferer may feel after leaving home can be allayed a little by frequent contact with a familiar person. The agitation may worsen temporarily at visits, but do not fall into the trap of thinking, 'Oh, she'll settle better if I don't come for a week. It will give her a chance to get used to people here.' This is sometimes suggested with the kindest of intentions by staff but is, frankly, cruel and thoughtless behaviour towards a person with a failing memory who cannot retain the image of a loved person in her mind for a long time and who needs frequent reminders to retain her identity as a family member.

After admission

Adjusting to life in a home takes time. Friends and relatives can play an important role in helping an elderly person to settle. The important notion to keep in mind is to help her remain one of the family and preserve her place in the past and present. The staff caring for her will be helped too if you take in mementoes, family photos, pictures of the relative on her wedding day, at work and in the family. Make sure the staff know *who* the resident is; not just her name, but her achievements, work, family background and so on. You can talk to the elderly person about what is happening in the family; even if it does not always seem to sink in or be remembered, she may just enjoy hearing the sound of your voice.

You do not have to talk when you visit, however. Just sitting in the same room while you do your knitting or writing can be reassuring to the resident. It is better to go for ten minutes three times a week than three deadly boring hours once a month. And don't just visit your own relative; speak to the other residents. You will find in any case that you get to know some of them and their families. If you can possibly help with voluntary activities in the home, fund-raising, outings, Christmas bazaars and so on, you will get to know the staff better, which may help the way you feel about the home.

Complaints

The following are the complaints most often made by residents' relatives to residential home staff:

- 'She's lost one/some/all of her best cardigans since coming in here.'
- 'Why doesn't her hearing-aid work?'

- 'Her spectacles have gone missing again.'
- 'Why didn't someone tell me when she fell and hurt herself?'
- 'She shouldn't have fallen over. You should be watching her.'
- 'She shouldn't be allowed out to wander round the streets. Why can't you keep the door locked?'
- 'She's not half so confused as these other people. Can't she be with less deteriorated people?'
- 'Can't you keep her away from that aggressive resident?'
- 'Why isn't she wearing one of her own dresses?'

It is not my intention to defend under all circumstances staff caring for elderly people, and staff are rightly expected to supervise and care for an elderly person to the best of their abilities. But remember, they have many residents to care for, not just one, and they cannot provide the kind of one-to-one care that you can give at home. Remember too that the confused people in the home will inadvertently pick up each other's belongings. Things get mislaid. Clothing that is frequently washed goes missing in the laundry. Incontinent elderly people need changing frequently; your mother may occasionally find herself wearing a borrowed dress because there are no more clean ones of her own. Wandering out will happen, and falls do occur; only superhuman powers of observation and mollycoddling the residents to the point of interfering with their physical freedom will prevent such incidents altogether.

Sometimes when relatives complain about trivial things they seem to be saying, 'I feel guilty because I couldn't look after the person better myself. I want to be extra sure that other people are doing the caring properly.'

Important issues to complain about are evidence of thoughtlessness or unkindness by the staff, an over-rigid regime, restrictive rules or a punitive attitude towards the confused or bad-tempered. If you get a whiff of anything like this affecting your relative, *complain fast*, to the manager, the proprietor or the registering body, the local authority social services or the district health authority.

Long-stay care in a psychiatric hospital

Individuals with severe behaviour disturbance, an inability to perform any personal care task without help or severe persistent incontinence may not be accepted by an old people's home or nursing home. The only option available may be a place in a ward for dementia sufferers in the local psychiatric hospital. 'Local' is often a misnomer; it is usually some miles away from the place where the elderly person resides.

Some of the liveliest and best psychogeriatric units are part of large psychiatric hospitals. The drive to develop specialist services for elderly dementia sufferers arose largely from psychiatrists working in wards of severely affected patients. A great deal has been done to improve the wards and maintain a good standard of care. However, these enormous institutions are not best designed to provide a homely environment, and the sometimes scandalously low levels of nurse staffing on the wards may mean that there is little time to do more than dress, feed, wash and toilet the patients. Staff morale is difficult to maintain in these circumstances, and the nursing management hierarchy tends to be set in entrenched, defensive ways that resist all change. The remarkable thing is how good ward nurses manage to do a fine caring job in spite of all these difficulties.

If your relative has to go into a long-stay ward of a psychiatric hospital, try to get involved with the ward and its activities. Get to know the sister or 'charge' nurse and the nursing aides caring for your relative. Relatives often feel angry on behalf of the staff at the mammoth task the nurses bear, and do not know how to agitate for better conditions for staff and patients. Write to the secretary of your community health council, your local councillor and your MP. Do as much agitating publicly as you can; patients cannot 'carry the baton' for themselves. None of us should end our days in an institution with inadequate care, and those of us who feel this way must make as loud a fuss as possible to ensure that there is better provision made for those in need.

Sheltered flats

Sheltered flats are blocks, usually of bed-sitting rooms or one-bedroom flats, where a warden lives on site and is available for emergency calls. There is usually an emergency alarm system. The warden may be assisted by deputies who do not live on site but help out for a few hours in the day. There is often a communal lounge for residents, and the warden may organise group activities once or twice a week. Many sheltered flats are owned by the local borough housing department, but there are also many private developments, especially in the retirement areas along the South Coast. As a general rule, sheltered flats are *not* suitable for elderly people with dementia. Even a mild degree of confusion makes living alone difficult, and the assistance provided by wardens is usually insufficient to provide adequate care. Wardens have little training in the needs of the frail elderly, are not nurses and do not generally perform personal care tasks. Meals-on-wheels and home helps may go in regularly, but the warden will perhaps call only once a day to see if all is well. The resident must be capable of using the emergency call system when she needs help quickly.

Many families are tempted to find a sheltered flat for a confused elderly person, hoping that a bright modern flat with a warden on site will be enough to provide the help and care the individual needs. A placement in sheltered flats can be disastrous for someone with dementia, particularly if they were barely coping in the familiar surroundings of their old home. They should either stay where they are, or alternatively live somewhere they can be supervised around the clock.

7

Finances and Legal Problems

It is often not recognised that dementia can pose a severe financial burden on the family of the sufferer. If the person suffering from dementia has to give up paid work as a result of the illness, the effect on the family income is obvious. More frequently, another member of the family who would otherwise be working has to give up work to care for the dementia sufferer. This person is often a married woman. The state gives less help on the whole to women, whom it assumes are not wage earners, than to men. On top of lost income, additional costs are incurred in providing extra light and heating, special clothing and equipment, incontinence aids, laundry bills, modifications to the home, extra transport costs for hospital or other appointments and so on. There may also be legal fees to pay or the cost of a sitter to find.

Help is available from the state for some of these expenses, but relatives frequently do not claim the welfare benefits that the sufferer and her supporters are entitled to. There are several reasons why benefits are not claimed. First there is a misconception that the whole family must be 'on the bread-line' before someone is entitled to help. This is not the case at all. An elderly person who is entitled to an attendance allowance, for example, may choose to give that allowance to her caring children to pay for her to have a private night sitter for one or two nights per week even if the children may not qualify for any special financial assistance because their income is deemed adequate. The second reason why benefits are not claimed is the uneasy feeling that benefits are charity hand-outs. It should be remembered that benefits paid to dependent people and their carers are payments from the national purse for which working people pay national insurance contributions throughout their adult lives. This elementary principle is not always grasped by elderly people themselves, who remember with distaste the prying 'means test' enquiries that preceded the meagre benefits of the 1930s. Thirdly, getting the right help from state resources is not always easy. The local social security office is usually a gloomy, unwelcoming place. Leaflets on different types of benefit are not always written in a way that can be easily understood. Filling in the application forms can be tedious and difficult for those unused to putting pen to paper. Fourthly, however, the major problem is simply that many people do not realise that they could get extra financial help if they applied.

Many people assume that the dementia sufferer who is better off, owns property and has a little money put by in a deposit account or building society poses few financial problems to relatives. The caring relative may nevertheless run into difficulties getting access to those financial resources because, even in the case of a married couple, accounts or property are often held solely in the sufferer's own name. Elderly people are sometimes unwilling to let someone else manage their affairs through lack of insight into their difficulties; alternatively they may be unable through loss of comprehension to transfer their affairs to someone else's management. Nevertheless there are ways of resolving these problems, provided you go about them in the right way.

Financial resources from the state

The first step is to find out what is available. You can get *social security leaflets* from the local social security office or perhaps more conveniently from the local post office. There is even a leaflet listing the leaflets (No. NI 146). A further source of information on benefits for pensioners is *Your Rights*, a booklet published annually by Age Concern. (See the Appendix for addresses.) The Citizens' Advice Bureaux also give advice on benefits and how to claim them. The following list of benefits comprises those that are most frequently forgotten. The government is currently reviewing the whole system of welfare benefits, so it is essential to get up-to-date information.

Supplementary pension

This is an extra amount of money paid to people whose income from other sources does not reach the level that the government considers necessary to live on. The level is reviewed each year. Social security staff calculate the individual's weekly income and weekly requirements and work out a figure appropriate for the individual. Special needs such as help with heating, insurance, repairs, laundry for incontinence, and travelling expenses for hospital treatment may be taken into account.

A person receiving supplementary pension may also be able to claim single payments to cover essential items such as clothing, bedding, furniture or removal expenses. The leaflets on supplementary pension and benefits are numbered SB 1, SB 16 and A 14N. *If in doubt, find out*.

Attendance allowance

A person who is severely disabled, either mentally or physically, and who has needed the attention of another person by day or by night, or both, for at least six months, can claim attendance allowance. The payment is made to the dependent person, not to the carer. The idea is that the individual can spend this extra money buying the services he or she requires. There is a lower rate paid to a person who needs attention either by night *or* by day, and a higher rate is paid to someone who needs twenty-four-hour attention. The attendance allowance can make an important contribution to the family income and is one of the most useful sources of state assistance to those who have become very dependent on others.

Leaflet NI 205 explains how to claim and has an application form (DS 2) attached. Make sure you attach a list of the real difficulties your relative has – for example, wandering at night, help required with bathing, using the toilet and dressing, risk of hurting herself if left because of forgetfulness, difficulty managing money. A doctor will be asked to visit the claimant to make an assessment and will of course need to talk to the relative about what the difficulties are. Elderly people with dementia can appear frustratingly alert and competent when the social security doctor calls; but the doctor should be aware of this. It is nevertheless important for a relative to give the true picture. If your claim is unsuccessful or your relative is offered the lower rate when you consider the higher rate more appropriate, you can appeal on behalf of your relative. A good number of reviews are successful.

Invalid care allowance

A man or woman below retirement age who spends at least thirty-five hours a week looking after someone who receives an attendance allowance can claim an invalid care allowance. The benefit is paid only to those who cannot work outside the home because of their caring commitments. The amount paid varies according to whether there are other dependants, such as children, to be provided for. The person receiving invalid care allowance is automatically credited with national insurance contributions so that later pension rights are not affected.

Until recently this benefit was only paid to men and single women. However, as a result of a decision in the European courts this benefit is now available to married women too. It is reckoned that the majority of younger people caring for dependent elderly relatives are married women, usually daughters or daughters-in-law. There are probably about 100,000 married women who stay at home to care for a sick person, many of whom would otherwise be able to go out to work. The majority of married women do now work outside the home. The unequal treatment of men and women was especially inappropriate at a time when the government wished to encourage 'care in the community'. Married women do most of the work at great personal cost, but until recently could receive no financial help from the state. The new ruling will go some way to redress the inequalities between the sexes.

Invalid care allowance guidelines and claim form are in leaflet NI 212.

Mobility allowance

This benefit seems to be designed to be of least help to those who need it most. Instead of the bias being against one sex, the bias this time is against one age group: old people. Mobility allowance is paid to severely disabled people to help them to become mobile, for example by hiring taxis or helping towards car expenses. The recipient must be virtually unable to walk because of physical disability. The 'catch 22' here is that the claimant must have become immobile before the age of sixty-five. The allowance can be claimed for up to twelve months after the person turns sixty-five and then it will continue until the person is seventy-five. The majority of severely disabled people are elderly but they do not qualify. Free bus passes are useless to this group of people, who need more help to get around. The age limit is a convenient but unfair method of restricting the amount of government spending on this particular benefit. A claim form is attached to leaflet NI 211.

Appeals

Yes, there is a leaflet (No 246) explaining how to appeal if you think the amount of benefit you or your relative is receiving is incorrect or that you have been wrongly refused a claim. You must appeal within twenty-eight days of the decision being made. Seek advice and try to get someone who knows the system to accompany you if you are going to an appeals tribunal. Your Citizens' Advice Bureau or legal aid centre can help you here.

Help while a person is in hospital

When an elderly person is admitted to hospital, assessment, treatment and rehabilitation often take longer than for a younger patient. The elderly person's home is often left unattended and in danger of decay through damp, vandalism and lack of maintenance. It is possible for the local authority to give financial and practical assistance to maintain the property in good order under Section 48 of the National Assistance Act. Contact the finance officer of the local social services department for information.

Someone receiving supplementary benefit may be able to claim back the cost of fares for travelling to and from hospital appointments and the cost of an essential escort's fares. There can also be help with travelling costs incurred in visiting a close relative in hospital.

If an elderly patient is in hospital for longer than eight weeks, their national insurance pension is reduced to a very small amount of 'pocket money', the assumption being that board and lodging are being provided by the National Health Service. A spouse remaining at home should immediately make enquiries about whether he or she is entitled to increased benefits to pay for those costs that may now be a problem as a result of this reduced income. It is another peculiar anomaly of our Welfare State that the only people who have to contribute financially to their care in hospital are elderly people, chronically disabled people and the unemployed.

Taking charge of a person's affairs

Someone who is mildly forgetful or just occasionally confused may be perfectly able to make rational judgements about their financial affairs and may merely need reminding to pay the bills on time and collect the pension. But a person with progressive dementia will eventually be unable to take legal or financial responsibility for their own affairs and will need someone to take charge. The elderly person is usually happy for someone else to collect the pension and pay the bills, and a relative or a trusted home help may take on this task without any other legal procedure being necessary. The problem arises when the individual's home needs to be sold or relatives want access to savings to pay for the larger bills or to meet nursing-home costs.

The answer does not lie in cajoling, persuading or charming the elderly person into signing documents that they do not understand. Signatures obtained under these circumstances are worthless.

The first step to take is to find a solicitor who can advise you on what plans you should make. He or she can advise you on how best to protect the interests of the confused person. If you do not know a solicitor, ask a friend or relative to recommend one or, failing that, write to the Law Society (113 Chancery Lane, London WC1), who can give you a list of local solicitors. When you meet the solicitor for the first time, explain the problem, find out about the fees he or she charges and also about whether he or she has experience of this kind of problem. If you are receiving supplementary benefits you may be entitled to legal aid to cover part or all of these costs. A list of solicitors who practise under the Legal Aid Scheme will be found in the local library or in the Citizens' Advice Bureau.

Power of attorney

A person who is mentally competent to manage his or her own affairs but is unable because of age, physical infirmity or other reasons to deal with the day-to-day transactions may give power of attorney to a spouse, adult child, friend or any other person to manage his or her finances and affairs. A power of attorney can be a general one, giving power to the named person to do whatever they feel appropriate; or it may be more specific and limited, e.g. to sell a particular property.

To give power of attorney, a person must be mentally competent and fully able to understand the nature and extent of the powers that she is investing in another person on her behalf. *An elderly person with dementia, confusion, paranoid illness or severe depression is not mentally competent to give power of attorney.* Furthermore, an existing power of attorney normally becomes automatically invalid if the person giving authority becomes mentally incompetent. However, a sensible alteration in the law has been introduced recently to allow an enduring power of attorney that will continue to operate when the person is no longer mentally competent. The signing over of powers must still be made while the individual is fully mentally alert.

The restrictions on power of attorney protect a mentally ill person from the possible greed of relatives. Unrestricted power of attorney gives a relative total freedom to do with the estate what he wishes. Although the person holding the power of attorney is legally responsible to do what is in the other person's best interests, there is wide scope for abuse.

Court of Protection

If an elderly person is unable through mental illness to manage her own affairs and has not given a valid power of attorney to someone else, then a relative (or professional person if there are no relatives) must apply to the Court of Protection for an order to appoint someone to act on behalf of the individual in order to administer her financial affairs. The person appointed by the court to act in this way, usually a spouse, relative or close friend, is called the *receiver*. If there is no one willing or able to act as receiver, then the court can appoint an official of the court. Applications to the court may be made by a solicitor or you can apply direct through the personal application branch of the court. The court charges a fee for administering someone's estate, unless it is a very small one. A Court of Protection order needs a medical certificate stating that the person is mentally incapable of managing her affairs. The solicitor is responsible for sending the forms to the family doctor or consultant who knows the patient. There is often a fee for the doctor's examination and certification included in the solicitor's bill.

From the relative's point of view, the court is a mixed blessing. The time between the application and the order being granted can be months, although the court is trying to speed things up. Spouses, in particular, often feel aggrieved that the home and savings which they have long felt to be theirs, even if by accident or by default they happen to be in their spouse's name, cannot be touched without getting permission from the court. A jointly owned marital home cannot be sold without a Court of Protection order. Furthermore, relatives resent having to pay the administration fees.

Although the vast majority of relatives have the best interests of the dependent person at heart and are willing to spend the individual's assets to provide good nursing care and comforts, there are less virtuous relatives who would let greed overcome their finer feelings. The court exists to protect the interests of the mentally ill person, not of their relatives. All the transactions that a caring relative would normally wish to carry out once they are appointed as receiver are usually acceptable to the court.

The Court of Protection publishes a number of leaflets on how it works and the role of a receiver. Write to it at 25 Store Street, London WC1E 7BP.

Authorisation procedures

If someone lives in rented accommodation and has little or no personal savings or other assets, it is not usually necessary to apply for a Court of Protection order. Benefits and pensions can be paid to a named appointee if the pension-book holder signs the correct part of the book. The DHSS may also give permission for the appointee to manage the pension on behalf of the individual, and the social security office will arrange this if appropriate. Private pensions can sometimes be handled in this way too, and it is worth enquiring of the former employer if this is possible. Small bank accounts are sometimes made available to spouses at the discretion of the bank manager, who will often ask for a letter of confirmation about the problem from a doctor. The bank manager may also be able to arrange a loan for a relative to cover living costs and expenditure incurred while a Court of Protection order is sought. In my experience, bank managers are generally very helpful and understanding in such cases; it really is worth discussing any financial problems with them.

Finding out what assets the elderly person has

Elderly people often have assets that they have forgotten about. Insurance policies taken out long ago, savings certificates, small numbers of shares or premium bonds are frequently left untouched when they could provide a little extra financial help. Hunting for evidence of assets requires detective work in obscure corners of the house. People really do keep money and important papers under carpets or beds, in biscuit tins or in even more bizarre places. You should look for evidence of bank accounts, building society accounts, share certificates, savings bonds, life insurance and health insurance policies, and retirement or disability benefits. A good look round will also reveal current debts in the shape of bills, loans, rate demands and so on. (Be prepared also for a possible surprise or two. Our elderly people were brought up in a much more rigid society. I know of two families who were shocked recently to turn up details of completely unknown half-brothers and half-sisters, in both cases the results of wartime liaisons that the parents chose not to discuss with the rest of the family.)

Testamentary capacity

In order to make a valid will a person must be mentally capable of understanding that she is making a will, must be able to make a rational judgement about the future disposal of her estate to named individuals and must have a knowledge of the extent of her assets. Being mentally competent to make a will is called having 'testamentary capacity'. In the very early stages of dementia it is possible for the impaired person to make or change a will, but it is essential that such a person is declared legally competent by an expert doctor. Even if the individual is found to be competent, relatives who persuade an easily led frail elderly person to change a will in their favour are in danger of being accused of bringing 'undue influence' to bear on the individual. If at all possible, therefore, avoid being involved with any changing of wills at this stage. When the person is no longer competent to make a will, as a result of dementia, or when rational judgement is affected by a paranoid illness or severe depression, any will made under these circumstances is invalid and could be challenged after the person's death. The best way to avoid problems like this is for all mentally competent individuals to make a will, with the help of a solicitor, earlier in life. Have *you* made a will? Now is the right time.

The Mental Health Act

This book is not the right place to debate the ethical issues surrounding the rights of elderly people with mental illness. The right to remain at home and at risk against the wishes of all those around often has to be balanced against other rights of mentally ill people to receive appropriate treatment and care in decent surroundings, compulsorily if necessary. Relatives are often very frustrated by the fact that their elderly relative cannot be forced to accept help, made to enter residential accommodation or removed against their will to hospital or a nursing home. When an individual's judgement and insight are impaired but she maintains that she is perfectly well and needs no help or alternative accommodation, there is no easy way to change the situation. However, the provisions of the Mental Health Act do allow for the compulsory admission to hospital and treatment of mentally ill people who are at risk of becoming seriously ill or of injuring themselves or who are placing others at risk.

The majority of patients 'sectioned' (i.e. compulsorily detained under Sections 2 or 3 of the Act) under the Mental Health Act are younger people suffering from reversible, treatable mental disorders who will recover and be discharged home quite quickly. Some elderly people suffering from depression, who are suicidal or at risk of starvation or dehydration and have become unable to think rationally, are compulsorily admitted to hospital for treatment. Patients with paranoid illnesses who pose a threat to themselves or to others are also sometimes compulsorily admitted. All these elderly patients will be discharged home when recovered.

Dementia sufferers pose a much greater problem in that the patient has an irreversible, final illness in which the individual may feel perfectly well and may much prefer to remain at home. 'Sectioning' such a person nearly always sentences her to long-term residential care in hospital or in an old people's home. Few psychiatrists and psychogeriatricians feel happy about using a compulsory Mental Health Act order to admit someone with dementia unless there are very grave risks to the patient of death from serious disease or injury or unless others, particularly caring relatives, are carrying a greater burden than can reasonably be expected. Relatives have rights too, to live without being physically abused or made ill by demented relatives.

Compulsory admission to hospital: how the Act works

A patient who is suffering from mental disorder that warrants assessment or treatment in hospital and ought to be admitted in the interests of her own health or safety, or with a view to the protection of others, may be compulsorily admitted for twenty-eight days if the person has refused voluntary admission. An *application* is usually made by a social worker with special training for this work but may also be made by the *nearest* blood relative. The social worker can act only if there are two medical recommendations. The two doctors, one of whom is usually the family doctor and the other a consultant psychiatrist or psychogeriatrician, must examine the patient. In practice, the family doctor or social worker usually initiates the 'section' procedure; and, if the view of all concerned is that compulsory admission is appropriate, the order is made and the patient is admitted to hospital. The entire procedure need take no more than a few hours.

If the patient is in need of treatment in hospital for longer than twenty-eight days, there is provision to detain her for up to six months. Elderly people often remain in hospital as voluntary patients after the expiry of the order, and it is unusual for orders to be extended for longer than six months. The patient does not necessarily remain in hospital for the full length of the order. The consultant will discharge the patient if she recovers with treatment. Sometimes the patient is willing to consider going to live in a residential home after a period in hospital when the inevitability of the need for institutional care is recognised and accepted.

In an emergency, a compulsory admission can be arranged by a social worker or relative on the recommendation of one doctor, but this should happen only very rarely. Compulsory admission to hospital is a bewildering, frightening and upsetting experience for anybody and especially distressing for a confused person who does not understand what is happening. On the other hand, it is more honest to take legal steps to commit someone to hospital rather than dishonestly to mislead people about 'going for an outing in the car', then abandoning them in the local hospital or residential home.

Guardianship

This is generally a rather better long-term solution to the problem of providing appropriate care for someone who has a long-standing mental disorder that prevents them from being able to care for themselves adequately.

The idea behind a guardianship order is that a close relative, or a social worker acting on behalf of the local authority if there are no suitable relatives, can act rather like a parent in relation to a child and exercise certain powers over a mentally disordered person who is unable to live without supervision. The powers of a guardian are not so wide or all-embracing as a parent's over a young child but they allow the guardian to determine where the individual should live, to insist that the individual attends for medical treatment or daily occupation as necessary and to insist that the person sees a visiting doctor or social worker. A guardian cannot insist that the patient *accepts treatment*, only that the individual *attends* for it. This may seem odd, but a person under a guardianship order still has the ability to refuse active medical treatment if she wishes.

A guardianship order is issued by the local authority. The application is made by the nearest relative or a specially trained social worker on the recommendation of two doctors, just like the compulsory admission orders. A guardianship order lasts for six months in the first instance but can be renewed as necessary.

The great advantage of a guardianship order is that it is less restrictive than a compulsory admission order and it allows times for decisions to be made in an unhurried way so that the person may be prepared to take an active part in the decisions being made. The following example shows how guardianship works:

Mr Beech was a 75-year-old widower who lived alone with his pet dog in a council house. He suffered from dementia and became increasingly unable to look after himself. He wandered out at night, left gas taps turned on but unlit, burnt out kettles and lived in some squalor. He refused to have any help in the house and was convinced that nothing was amiss. He accepted meals-on-wheels but gave them to his dog. Meanwhile he ate little and became thinner, paler and listless. Mr Beech's only daughter lived some miles away and could not do more than make regular visits, do a little shopping and try to persuade him to eat. It became clear that Mr Beech was at serious risk of falling ill, but he refused to consider residential care. His daughter applied for a guardianship order on the recommendation of his GP and the local psychogeriatrician. His social worker helped the daughter to find an appropriate residential home where Mr Beech could take his dog and preserve his privacy in a room of his own. It took three months to find the right place, and Mr Beech was well prepared for the move and visited the home on several occasions beforehand. He was still reluctant to move but able to understand that the order was compulsory. Six months later Mr Beech, looking fit and well, was settled and able to say he liked his new home and intended to stay. The guardianship order was then allowed to expire.

A guardian does not have the power to use the individual's money or assets or to manage her financial or legal affairs. The guardian must apply to the Court of Protection in the usual way to take charge of the finances.

Guardianship orders are used less than they should be. Local authorities have not always been happy to take on the extra duties and responsibilities of administering these orders. This is a great pity as they serve a very useful function in protecting an elderly person with dementia from severe self-neglect and in giving proper authority to a near relative to provide appropriate care.

Section 47 of the National Assistance Act

This section is not a part of the Mental Health Act but is a much older provision that is little used nowadays. In effect it allows for the compulsory removal from their homes to a hospital or residential home of two sorts of people: those who are suffering from serious physical illness and old people who are living in insanitary squalor. Both these groups are eligible for removal if they are not able to look after themselves properly and are a risk to themselves or a risk to others. A magistrate issues the order on the recommendation of a public health doctor, supported by another medical recommendation. This old-fashioned act is very rarely used because there are other more appropriate ways of dealing with the problems of mentally ill old people, and those who are mentally well are usually considered able to make their own decisions on whether to accept treatment or residential care.

8

Mental Health Problems Associated with Physical Illness in Elderly People

Elderly people are much more likely than younger people to suffer from physical illness and to be handicapped by a wide range of disabilities. Even those relatively fit elderly people who regard themselves as being generally in good shape are likely to be troubled by hearing and sight defects or by a spot of rheumatism or indigestion. A number of diseases become much more common in old age. This is because the ageing process itself can produce problems and also because illnesses can be the consequence of a particular way of life. Our diet, the exercise we take, our smoking and drinking habits, even the jobs we do can all affect our health, and these health problems generally manifest themselves in old age. Chest and heart disease, diabetes, strokes, arthritis, Parkinson's disease, deafness and poor sight are all increasingly common with advancing age.

It is beyond the scope of this book to consider in depth this wide range of problems. However, some of these common conditions frequently give rise to mental health problems, which create difficulties for relatives caring for an elderly person at home. This chapter covers the commoner problems arising as a consequence of physical illness.

How can you tell when an old person is physically ill?

Illness often starts in elderly people in an unusual and undramatic fashion. For example, a heart attack is usually a very dramatic event in a middle-aged person, manifested by a constricting chest pain, a shocked grey face and a feeling of clamminess and dizziness. An elderly person by contrast can have a 'silent coronary' that is totally painless but gives rise to mental confusion and falls. The absence of specific symptoms is common to diseases in old age. Instead of clear physical symptoms pointing to the origin of the problem, less obvious and more general signs of illness are present instead. Confusion, unsteadiness, sudden immobility ('She's gone off her feet') and urinary incontinence are symptoms that tell us *something* is physically wrong, but they may not necessarily point to the exact cause. These symptoms are always worth reporting to the doctor, who can then enquire more closely into the problem.

Acute confusional states

An acute confusional state is a condition in which mental confusion begins suddenly. Another name for an acute confusional state is *delirium*. Most people's idea of delirium is probably the rambling confusion of a fever-racked, semi-conscious hero of an action-packed adventure film. In real life delirium is rarely like that. In its mildest forms it can be very hard to diagnose and in its more severe forms can be a bewilderingly chameleon-like condition, changing symptoms from hour to hour.

Acute confusional states can mimic dementia (for the difference between the two, see below). It is easy to misdiagnose a person as having dementia if a clear account of the illness is not available. This can be catastrophic because acute confusional states are treatable, and in the majority of cases full recovery will occur.

Delirium can occur at any age when someone is seriously ill and is particularly associated with a high temperature and fever. Elderly people and young children are especially liable to become confused when ill. Mothers take in their stride the confused and nonsensical utterings of unwell children and refer to mild confusion as 'rambling' or 'feverishness', but we do not expect adults to react in the same way. Confusion in elderly people can be perplexing and sometimes frightening but is really the same thing.

Acute confusional states are the result of a physical upset to the body affecting the normal functioning of the brain, reducing the brain's capacity to think, reason and perceive clearly. The underlying physical cause can be one of a wide range of problems such as infections, transient strokes or too much medication or alcohol. The commonest causes in elderly people are mentioned below.

What is an acute confusional state like?

Confusion begins very suddenly, usually over the course of twenty-four hours. Someone can be completely normal one day and utterly confused the next. *Dementia does not start like this at all*; it develops slowly, usually over a matter of months. In an acute confusional state there are usually wide swings in the severity of confusion ranging from a slightly perplexed mood and mild forgetfulness to profound dis-orientation, sleepiness and an inability to communicate. These swings can occur in just an hour or two. This changeability makes it very difficult to tell is someone is getting better or not, since one day may be symptom-free, and the person may appear to have returned to her alert old self, but this may then be followed by a disturbing night of confusion.

Confusion is shown by impaired mental grasp and by forgetfulness and disorientation. The person does not realise where she is, who is with her or what time of day it is. She has difficulty concentrating and understanding what is said to her. Conversation tends to be slow and disjointed, with the individual missing entirely what is said to her.

The person usually appears *perplexed and anxious*, troubled by the experience. Sometimes she appears to be in a dream-like state or self-preoccupied daze. On the other hand, the mood can change quickly to one of agitation, anger and frightened suspicion.

The person suffering from confusion or delirium does not lie 'Hollywood style', tossing and turning in bed, but is almost always *agitated*, *restless* and wanting to be up and about, on the go. In the middle of the night confused individuals often get up and wander around the house, knocking over obstacles. The inability to stay still can be very upsetting in a general hospital ward or in an old people's home where everyone else gets less sleep when a disturbed patient rambles around in a confused state. Some people repeatedly carry out actions such as drinking a cup of invisible tea or dusting the furniture with an invisible duster as if they were living through a dream or repeating some daily task as a habit.

Visual illusions are very common. Perhaps the most usual problem encountered is seeing moving patterns on the carpet or wallpaper, often misinterpreted as animals or insects. Shadows may appear as figures. Sometimes 'people' appear in the room who look realistic to the patient but are often curiously smaller than usual, so that the person observes the apparitions as children or dwarfs. These visual problems are compounded by poor eyesight caused by cataracts and glaucoma and are often made worse by gloomy lighting and at night-time. More unusually, sounds of voices, music and bells may be heard, or conversations imagined. When visual illusions or hallucinations are experienced for hours at a time out of the blue by a person who was previously mentally alert, there is always an underlying cause. The individual should be examined, and the problem should be investigated, by a doctor.

Delusions. We have already mentioned delusional or false ideas in Chapter 3 and will be talking more fully about them in Chapter 10. Mistaken ideas of being persecuted or harmed are very common in acute confusional states but tend to fluctuate and change from hour to hour. Often the patient is unable to describe her feelings accurately but behaves in a terrified way, trying to get away from other people and reacting with frightened belligerence to those trying to nurse her. These ideas sometimes lead the individual mistakenly to try to 'escape', for example by climbing out of a window.

The person usually looks *ill*. She often has a rapid pulse, falls about in a dizzy state, looks flushed and tremulous. However, some people seem to muster the strength of Hercules even when suffering in this way and are extremely difficult to nurse as a result of their over-activity and restlessness, rejecting the helping hands and pleas to rest from those around them.

How long will the confusion last?

If the underlying cause of the problem is treated promptly, a patient with confusion may recover within a few days. Recovery is usually a jerky affair, one good day followed by a bad and then followed by a good day again, but the confused episodes normally disappear altogether eventually. However, confusion can carry on for a week or two and much longer than that in some cases. For example, after a stroke, when the brain is adjusting to the sudden illness, a patient may be forgetful and confused for six weeks or more but then recover completely.

Doctors and nurses tend to feel that their treatments cannot be working if confusion continues for a while after they have begun the treatment. But the brain takes a while to adjust itself again, and often professionals and relatives have to be patient to let the confused person recover in their own good time.

When the patient has recovered, the events of the illness are usually completely forgotten, leaving a period of 'blank nothingness' while they were confused. Just occasionally, however, a frightening vision or imaginary episode may be remembered as if it were a reality, and it can be difficult to convince the person that the events did not really happen.

Common causes of acute confusional states

Any physical condition that upsets the body's delicate metabolic balance can cause an acute confusional state. The cause is usually not too difficult to identify if the patient has a pre-existing condition that has worsened recently. For example, an elderly man with chronic bronchitis who develops a worse cough, with green phlegm, may well develop confusion as a result of the infection in the lungs. The cause is not always so obvious; blood tests and X-rays may be needed to diagnose the underlying problem.

The following physical conditions are those that are most commonly found affecting elderly people living at home and therefore most likely to lead to acute confusional states.

Chest infection

A bad chest, a worsening cough, a flu-like illness or a very bad cold are all very common causes of sudden confusion. The phlegm is often a nasty green colour, and the chest sounds noisier than usual. The person is often a smoker with long-standing chest problems and a tendency to get breathless. Elderly people do not necessarily develop high temperatures with a chest infection, but a doctor can usually detect the problem by listening to the lungs with a stethoscope.

Infections in the bladder

Most women have heard of *cystitis*, or infection in the urine, and a great many women have experienced it. A frequent urge to pass urine and an unpleasant burning sensation on voiding urine are the usual symptoms. Elderly people, however, can develop a urinary infection without any obvious symptoms. They do not necessarily experience the burning sensation or frequency, yet they often become suddenly and inexplicably unable to hold their water. This sudden incontinence is often accompanied by an unpleasant fishy smell to the urine, which clings to the person and her clothing. The combination of sudden confusion, incontinence, smelly urine and being generally unwell are pointers to the diagnosis.

Infection in leg ulcers and pressure sores

As we age, the blood circulation to our legs becomes less efficient. Small abrasions and bruises tend to become ulcers, especially on the ankles where the skin and tissues are tender and do not heal easily. Ulcers become infected very easily, and cellulitis, an inflammation of the skin and surrounding tissues, can develop quickly. The skin appears shiny, tense and reddened, and the surrounding flesh gets swollen and painful. Infection from these sources can lead to confusion. It may also occur as a result of infected pressure sores on heels and buttocks in an immobile elderly person.

Medication

All drugs can cause confusion if taken in the wrong doses. Perhaps the commonest ones to beware of are *sleeping tablets*, especially nitrazepam (Mogadon) and diazepam (Valium). The tablets have a cumulative effect on elderly people so that the level in the blood stream may still be quite high during the day following taking a sleeping-pill, and symptoms may therefore worsen as a result of medication every night.

Tablets taken to treat anxiety, nervousness and depression may also cause confusion. The dose of all these drugs has to be monitored very carefully by the prescribing doctor.

Sudden withdrawal of sedative drugs is also likely to cause confusion. Nitrazepam (Mogadon) is a common offender again, but lorazepam (Ativan) is also a likely culprit. Old-fashioned barbiturate sleeping-drugs like amylobarbitone (sodium amytal) and phenobarbitone are particularly liable to cause problems if stopped suddenly. If your relative is used to taking medication regularly, *never* stop the medication suddenly; always consult the doctor who prescribes them if you think the tablets may be contributing to confusion.

Alcohol

Drunkenness is a variety of acute confusional state most of us have witnessed (or experienced!) at one time or another. Elderly people can become confused and appear drunk after taking a relatively small amount of alcohol. This is because as we age our tolerance of alcohol decreases. Even when someone has been used to consuming several glasses of alcohol daily for many years, a time may come when they can hold very little alcohol without becoming confused, liable to fall and at risk of hurting themselves. Alcohol does not mix well with a lot of medications, and it is often the *combination* of tablets and drink that causes the problem.

Transient stroke

More details of what a stroke is and how it affects the mental processes are given later in this chapter. When someone has had an obvious stroke, leaving them weak down one side or with difficulty in speaking, no one will be very surprised if they become confused in the days or weeks following. It is however possible to have a small stroke with the results lasting only a few minutes or hours that leaves no permanent weakness or other obvious problems except mental confusion. A clue to the cause is if there was a fall or blackout or some evidence of weakness in an arm or leg. Sometimes the person just has an hour or two of difficulty in speaking or a short period of profound dizziness.

If the individual has had an earlier stroke or transient stroke then this is the most likely cause of a sudden onset of confusion. Confusion due to stroke can take several weeks to settle down. The person does not always return completely to their former alert self but may be left with some mental impairment.

How to tell confusion from dementia

Dementia begins slowly; acute confusion begins suddenly. Dementia sufferers vary from day to day but never return to their old selves in their alertness and competence, whereas in confusion the mental state can fluctuate dramatically from hour to hour and day to day. Someone who is confused often looks ill, while a dementia sufferer may appear physically quite well.

Dementia and acute confusion can occur together

Elderly people are liable to develop an acute confusional state when they become physically ill. But to complicate matters further, someone who has already developed a dementing illness is even more likely to develop symptoms of a confusional state if they become physically ill or are overmedicated. When someone with dementia gets *very much worse* within a few hours or days, then it is likely to be due to a physical illness upsetting the patient. Diagnosis is of course always made more difficult if the patient cannot describe what the problem is; a physical examination, blood tests and X-rays may be needed to detect the problem. Ask the doctor to call promptly when you suspect that delirium is developing on top of a dementia.

Helping the confused person

What should a relative do to help an elderly person with an acute confusional state? First, consult your family doctor as a matter of urgency. If the cause of confusion is obvious to you, *tell him*. You can save the doctor a lot of work. Second, if the cause can be treated at once, for example by antibiotic drugs, then if possible nurse your relative at home. When someone is confused, admission to hospital can be a frightening and upsetting experience. If you cannot manage the nursing because of ill health or because the person is seriously disturbed and frightened, ask the doctor to arrange for them to be admitted to hospital.

The patient should be admitted to a general hospital, to a specialist geriatric medical hospital or to a psychogeriatric assessment unit in a general hospital. *Resist* strongly any move to admit your relative to a mental hospital, because the facilities there for medical investigations and treatment are usually very poor.

In Britain, especially in areas where there is pressure on hospital beds, elderly people who are physically ill and mentally confused at the same time are more likely to be refused admission to hospital than other patients in serious need. This is very unfair and a sad reflection on our health service. The reasons are easy to understand, however. The medical staff fear that the person will become a 'bed blocker', someone who can never be discharged home because of severe mental and physical disability. Furthermore, few young doctors are trained to distinguish confusion from dementia and medical staff may therefore not always spot the underlying physical problem. This is where a relative's story can be so useful in stressing the sudden recent onset of the problem. Make sure that you accompany your relative to hospital so that you can give a full history to the staff; they won't know if you don't tell them.

Managing an elderly person with confusion at home

Acute confusion is an unpredictable and perplexing condition. Just when the person seems to have settled down to a good night's sleep, she wakes up and appears intent on spending the night roaming round the house. She is unable to listen to what is said to her and very often ignores those around her.

The key to managing a person at home is to stay as cool as possible. Keep reminding yourself that the symptoms are just the result of the illness and will soon settle down. Keep the lights bright, even at night if your relative is awake, and keep reminding her who you are and what you are doing. Do not worry too much whether or not she is eating properly but ensure that she drinks enough plain water, weak orange squash, mild or warm weak tea. The fluid will help keep her well hydrated. Do not give Lucozade or fizzy soft drinks such as Coca Cola or lemonade because they are too strongly laden with sugar and salts to be properly refreshing.

Sedative drugs are occasionally necessary to allay agitation and restlessness but should be used very sparingly since they may make the individual over-drowsy and mask the signs of recovery. Do not despair if the first medicine the doctor prescribes does not seem to help; the dose may need adjusting or the medication changing. Individuals respond very differently to different medicines, and it is often a matter of trial and error to find the right one.

Strokes

What is a stroke?

When the blood supply to part of the brain is disturbed, a stroke may occur. For example, the blood supply may be cut off because a small artery has burst and bled into the surrounding brain tissue. Alternatively, a clot or piece of debris floating round the arterial system can block up one of the small arteries and starve the nearby brain tissue of the oxygen that is carried in the arterial blood. The medical term for a stroke is *cerebro vascular accident*, a term that relatives sometimes find puzzling because they don't remember an 'accident'. However, it is the artery that has suffered the accident, not the patient. A stroke is a natural illness in just the same way as a coronary is.

Strokes may be very mild and transient with full recovery occurring within a few hours, but the effects are usually longer lasting. Depending on which side of the brain is affected and which area is deprived of blood, one side of the body becomes paralysed. The arm and leg become useless, and feeling is lost down that side. Sight and speech may also be affected. Sometimes the ability to think clearly and understand other people's speech is impaired.

What happens to the person's mental abilities?

It is important to realise that a stroke does not usually cause persistent confusion or dementia. The individual may think more slowly for a few weeks or months and often finds concentrating difficult, but any serious confusion usually resolves itself within a short time. Someone who has lost the ability to translate what she is thinking into audible speech may appear particularly confused, even when her thought processes may not really be confused at all. The loss of speech function can vary from merely a mild mixing up of words or a difficulty in finding the right word to a much more serious total loss of the ability to form any words. This is extremely frustrating and distressing for patients who know what they want to say but cannot get it out. Even worse is the loss of ability to comprehend the words spoken to the person. For example, if a person who has suffered a stroke is told to put out a hand in front of her she may understand a part of what is said and look in a puzzled way at her hand or try to stick out a foot instead.

Most of the disabilities improve with time. A relative can help enormously by being patient and by helping the sufferer to practise the right words. Some people find it useful to have a set of cards with pictures of common items on them so that they can show you what they want, e.g. pictures of a cup of tea, glass of squash, lavatory, electric heater and so on.

Emotional changes

The commonest emotional problem after a stroke is *depression*. As many as one in five of stroke victims become withdrawn, sad and lose their appetites. There is a strong temptation to say, 'Well, it's understandable, given how disabled the person is'; but we know that this kind of depression is much commoner after a stroke affecting the left side of the body than after a right-hand-side stroke. This suggests that the depression is due partly to the brain disturbance itself and not just to the patient's reaction to the stroke. Depression is often helped by the right medication. Because it prevents the stroke victim from making the effort required to get moving again and can have a serious effect on the final outcome, it is important to have the depression treated.

The other common emotional problem after a stroke, which can occur also in those with several transient, minor strokes, is *emotional lability*. This is sudden outbursts of tearfulness that come 'out of the blue' and are not clearly related to upsetting events. These outbursts can be very puzzling for the individual because weeping is not always accompanied by upsetting feelings. The weeping occurs suddenly and unpredictably. Some people also have outbursts of laughter and 'silliness', which can be equally embarrassing and distressing.

It is easy to confuse emotional lability with depression. The way to tell the difference is to *ask* the person to describe how she feels and to note whether sleep and appetite are affected and whether there is persistent unhappiness and pessimistic thoughts. A relative can help professionals to decide whether the main problem is true depression or emotional lability. Depression can be helped by medication, but emotional lability cannot be treated – although it usually improves over time.

A stroke can also affect a person's *motivation*. Some patients become curiously apathetic and listless, unconcerned about their profound disability and lacking in motivation to persist with exercises or tasks designed to speed function. Such individuals are usually happy enough; but family and professionals feel they are lazy and not trying hard enough, and feel frustrated that physiotherapy and occupational therapy are making no impact. Everyone feels cross with the person and expects far more in the way of improvement than is actually achieved. But it is not fair to blame the patient, who cannot help the fact that the loss of motivation and inertia is caused by the stroke damage to the brain. Pushing and cajoling will achieve nothing, except to get you upset.

Helping someone with a stroke

Write to the Chest, Heart and Stroke Association (see the Appendix for addresses) for leaflets on the effects of stroke and how to cope with them. Some districts have *stroke clubs*, which some patients and their relatives find useful. Your GP or the social worker attached to the hospital where your relative was first treated will know whether there is a club in your district.

Recovery is a gradual process taking months. The patient easily becomes discouraged when improvement is scarcely noticeable from one day to the next. Keep reminding them of what has been achieved since the first day.

Parkinson's disease

What is Parkinson's disease?

Most people have heard of this disease but often have mistaken ideas about the causes, the effects and what will happen to the sufferer. It is not a paralysing or wasting illness, and with modern treatment most patients can continue to live a full and enjoyable life for many years.

The disease is named after James Parkinson, a family doctor who practised in the East End of London in the early part of the nineteenth century. He described the illness in great detail, calling it 'the shaking palsy'. Parkinson's is a disease of a small part of the brain that controls the co-ordination of movement and balance. The proper function of this area of the brain depends on a balance between certain brain chemicals. In Parkinson's disease the brain cells are deficient in one of these chemicals, *dopamine*. We do not know exactly why this dopamine deficiency develops but it is commoner in middle-aged and older people.

Parkinson's is a progressive disease in that symptoms get gradually worse as the years go by. The rate of progression varies enormously from one patient to another, and effective treatment can control the symptoms for a long time.

Symptoms of Parkinson's disease

Tremor. The tremor of Parkinson's disease is worst when the patient is resting. One side is usually worse than the other and is best seen in the hands and fingers when the arms are resting on the lap. It is a rhythmic, noticeable shaking (not a 'vibration'), which disappears during sleep and is much diminished by purposeful movement. Holding a cup and saucer or reading a newspaper may appear to diminish the tremor. However, nervous tension and embarrassment make the tremor much worse; patients frequently become self-conscious about their shaking. It is often the self-consciousness and embarrassment caused by the tremor that deter the Parkinsonian patient from venturing out in public.

Stiffness. A patient with Parkinson's has stiff, rigid muscles that do not relax easily. The increased muscle tension is often felt as aches and pains and fatigue rather than as stiffness. The muscles of the face remain stiff and give the sufferer a rather blank, expressionless appearance. Sometimes the limbs feel heavy; one patient described the feeling as like the stiffness one feels getting out of bed the day after an unaccustomed bout of exercise.

Slow movement. Human beings normally move their muscles all the time. Even when sitting relaxed watching the television, our limbs move quite frequently; we alter our facial expressions, turn our heads, cross our legs and so on. Patients with Parkinson's have difficulty starting movements, and all movements become much slower than usual. Getting up from a chair, walking, using muscles of speech to talk, swallowing, making facial expressions all become slow and difficult to implement. Parkinson's patients tend to sit completely still with the flat expressionless face mentioned above. We depend so much on facial expression to understand what someone is feeling and thinking that it is difficult at first for relatives and friends to understand that the mental agility and liveliness of the patient's mind are preserved behind this depressed and rather uninterested-looking face. We must keep reminding ourselves that the patient's true feelings are not showing.

Slowing down also means that patients have to do *everything slowly, from dressing in the morning to cooking and going out on errands*. Other people tend to attribute this slowing to old age or mental infirmity. Like people in wheelchairs or those who have had strokes, most Parkinson's sufferers will have experienced being treated like imbeciles because of other people's lack of understanding that the problems are physical, not mental.

Getting started and coming to a halt are sometimes problematic. Some sufferers have particular difficulty initiating movement and have to wait a second or two before starting to walk. But once started, the legs tend to run away with themselves, going too quickly for comfort. One woman patient described this as 'like when I put my foot down too hard on my electric sewing-machine and the stitches overrun all over the place even after I've released the pedal'. These problems can be helped by having the right sort of walking-aid, but it does need a trained therapist to decide which aid is the right one for each individual. An aid with wheels may be just the thing for a 'difficult starter' but may make an 'overrunner' feel as if they are in a runaway train. So get expert advice when acquiring a walking-frame.

Disturbance of balance. Slowness and difficulty in co-ordinating movement lead to difficulties in maintaining an upright posture. Standing on one leg to step over something, going upstairs, stepping over a doorstep or getting on to a bus are all risky moments when the muscles may fail to co-ordinate properly. The sufferer may find herself flat on the floor, unable to get up. Few things are as embarrassing as ending up on the floor in a crowded public place, and even the *fear* of this makes people lose confidence and become increasingly housebound or chairbound.

Constipation. Reduced physical activity and a slowing of the bowel movements lead to constipation, which is often made considerably worse by medication. This distressing problem can be kept under control by the right high-fibre diet and 'bulk' laxatives. Taken regularly these have a beneficial effect on the activity of the bowel.

Dribbling. The Parkinson's sufferer appears to produce too much saliva, which dribbles out of the mouth embarrassingly. In fact we all produce just as much saliva, but normal people swallow frequently so it does not collect in the mouth. Sitting with the head up or tilted slightly back helps the saliva to drain away down the gullet naturally.

Skin problems. Parkinson's disease is often accompanied by greasy, scaly skin. Hair often develops dandruff, and the individual finds she sweats a lot. These curious symptoms, reminiscent of adolescent skin problems, are helped by using the special soaps recommended for teenagers with acne and by anti-dandruff shampoos. Women may find astringent lotions and the ranges of cosmetic products developed for teenagers useful.

Mental disorder associated with Parkinson's disease

Parkinson's disease is usually accompanied by a feeling of tiredness and a loss of energy. Everything is a great effort. The physical disability of course means that doing everyday chores *is* a great effort. Sufferers often feel too that they need more sleep than usual.

Depression, of the more serious kind described in Chapter 9, is common with the disease. Because the illness is so self evidently a disabling, distressing condition, relatives often dismiss the depression as an understandable response, which therefore does not require treatment. But depressive illness in Parkinson's disease is often the kind of depression that responds very well to the right medication. Gloomy ideas, pessimism, loss of appetite, weight loss and insomnia are all pointers to the kind of depression that can benefit from treatment. Patients often need a lot of encouragement to seek help for depression. They wrongly feel they are to blame for not coping better or pulling themselves together.

Memory problems. Most people with Parkinson's disease go on for many years without any difficulty whatever in remembering, concentrating or thinking clearly. However, after some years of illness a proportion of sufferers experience problems in recalling names, facts and incidents from the recent past. A curious and irritating symptom, which mirrors similar 'stop-start' physical problems, is that thoughts just suddenly seem to stop dead. We have all experienced interference with concentration so that we forget what to say next, but this kind of 'thought block' is different. It feels as if all thinking has suddenly been rubbed out of the mind and the thinker's brain has been wiped clean, just like wiping off a recording from a tape-recorder. This irritating symptom is of little significance in itself and certainly does not mean that the person's mind is going. There is unfortunately no treatment for it. The sufferer just has to accept it as an irritating fact of life.

Some patients with advanced Parkinson's disease have increasing problems with concentration, memory and progressive dementia. These can be similar to the problems of Alzheimer's disease described in Chapters 2 and 3.

Treatment

When Parkinson's disease was untreatable, patients succumbed to the physical disability and often did not live long enough for the more complex failure of the brain to become evident. Doctors are now seeing more patients survive with their physical problems under control but suffering from dementia. The effects of Parkinson's disease, coupled with the effects of medication and the influence of dementia and confusion, can be extremely difficult even for specialist doctors to disentangle. It can be very hard to sort out exactly what is causing which symptom. Professionals can jigger around with medication, physiotherapy and the right environment to help the patient function at her optimum, but sufferers and their relatives have to be very patient and observant to enable the doctors to find the best treatment. This treatment may need adjusting every few weeks or months, and you should ask your GP to recommend a specialist if things do not seem to be going well. Neurologists, geriatricians and psychogeriatricians all have plenty of experience in treating Parkinson's disease, which is nevertheless a very complicated mental disorder.

Medication for Parkinson's disease. There are two major groups of drugs used to treat Parkinson's disease. One group, called *anticholinergics*, has been around since the 1940s and these drugs are still used to treat the rigidity and tremor in mild cases. Benzhexol (Artane) and orphenadrine (Disipal) are two commonly prescribed drugs in this group. However, these drugs have now been largely superseded by drugs that replace or enhance the deficient brain chemical dopamine. Levodopa was the first dopamine-replacing drug and was discovered in the early 1960s. There are now a number of synthetic drugs suitable for some patients. The commonest dopamine-enhancing drugs prescribed at present are Sinemet, Madopar, Parlodel and Eldepryl.

Advances in medication inevitably bring with them unwanted side-effects and long-term complications. On the whole, the benefits far outweigh the disadvantages for most patients, but it is as well to be aware of the possible side-effects as these can so easily be mistaken for the symptoms of the illness. This can lead to a misguided attempt to 'treat' the symptoms by increasing the amount of the drug, the real cause of the problem.

Nausea, weight loss, unwanted abnormal movements of the face, arms and legs, cramps and a sudden switching on and off of the effect of the drug are all common side-effects. But the degree to which they are present varies widely. More unusual mental effects of dopamine-enhancing drugs are suspiciousness, obvious confusion, paranoid ideas and hallucinations. Sometimes a full-blown acute toxic confusional state develops (as described earlier) or a mental illness that is indistinguishable from the paranoid states described in Chapter 10. These symptoms are very distressing for both the patient and her relatives and need to be carefully evaluated by a specialist. Such symptoms *can* be treated, and it is rare for them not to be controlled when the patient is on the right individual course of drugs.

The Parkinson's Disease Society (see the Appendix) publishes a range of helpful booklets and lists of its local branches. Its newsletter will tell you about helpful books to give you more information.

Managing physical disability where mental disorder is also a problem: aids for living

This chapter cannot discuss in depth all the common physical illnesses that affect elderly people. Immobility because of arthritis, unsteadiness, persistent falls, breathlessness and pain are common enough symptoms in old age. All these symptoms deserve proper medical attention and are not just the inevitable consequence of growing old. Beware of any doctor who says, 'It's just old age', especially where physical illness and mental disorder go hand in hand. Some doctors find this difficult combination of conditions rather daunting and they are sometimes less eager to help than if the patient were younger and mentally alert. So you may have to press for a thorough examination and a second opinion if necessary.

Even with the best medical and remedial help, many elderly people suffer from serious physical handicaps which are wearing and distressing for the individual and physically taxing and tiring for those who nurse her. This is where *aids for living* come in. These are gadgets, equipment, machinery and furniture that are especially designed to enable a person to live a normal life, as far as possible. There are literally thousands of specially designed aids, but *many of them are not suitable for people who suffer from mental confusion or dementia*. This is because people usually have to learn to use an aid; new habits are acquired with practice, and mentally frail elderly people find this particularly hard. So *consult an expert* and reassure yourself that the aid will be used properly by the elderly person before borrowing or buying it.

Who provides and pays for such aids? This depends on where you live and who is recommending the aid. The National Health Service and some social services departments will provide aids on loan free of charge. Any aid for independent living may in theory be provided by the local social services departments at their discretion, if the money to buy it is available and if it has been recommended by an occupational therapist specifically employed to advise on aids. In many parts of Britain, however, the waiting-list is up to two years long for an initial visit by an occupational therapist; there is then a further wait for the council employees to come and fit the aid in the home or for it to be ordered from the manufacturer. All this can take a ridiculously long time, and meanwhile the poor sufferer has to do as best she can. Some local authorities have speeded up the process, and in some lucky areas people do not have to wait at all. To find out about the situation in your area, contact the occupational therapist, the adviser to the disabled or the rehabilitation therapist in your local social services department.

Aids are not always supplied free of charge; some councils make a charge according to the client's financial circumstances. It may be quicker to consult a professional adviser and pay for the aids and the installation yourself if this is within your means. *But do go to an independent adviser.* The manufacturer or shopkeeper who stocks only one or two kinds of aid has a vested interest in selling his own products.

The best source of advice in Britain is from the Disabled Living Foundation (see the Appendix for the address and telephone number). This charitable foundation provides an information service, leaflets on a host of different aids and lists of aids centres throughout the country where you can see and try out aids and equipment. If you live near enough to London you can phone for an appointment to discuss exactly what aids would be helpful for you and your relative's handicaps. You can also get information from a growing number of local advice centres. You can get their addresses from Dial UK Ltd (see the Appendix).

Examples of useful aids

Armchairs. Elderly people usually find a high-seated wing-chair or chair with padded arms more supportive and comfortable than a low chair. Wing-chairs also keep out drafts round the neck. You can have chairs raised on blocks or have extra footstools and cushions. Chairs with self-lifting seats are *not* very good for the mentally frail; being unexpectedly tipped out of a seat when you lean forward can be quite a shock. Some hospital chairs tip the patient up so they rest more comfortably, but the poor patient is left staring at the ceiling all day. Never use a tray attached across the chair to keep the person sitting down; this will cause feelings of imprisonment, and they may well hurt themselves trying to get out of the restraining chair.

Personal care and toilet. The floor of a toilet should be non-slip. A grab-rail is useful. If the toilet is too low a raised seat can be bought quite cheaply. If the toilet is upstairs or difficult to get to, then social services can provide a commode, which should be stable and not too low.

Getting in and out of the bath can be made easier by grab-rails on the wall, a pole hanging from a chain and a non-slip bath mat. More elaborate electrically operated hoists are also available. Showers are a lot easier than baths, but mentally frail elderly people who have never used them before may find them frightening and unpleasant.

Eating. A plate-guard or a specially designed plate will help with scooping up food. A non-slip mat under the plate will stabilise it. There is also specially designed cutlery for eating with one hand. Drinking-aids and bibs are available; but when choosing them, ask yourself if this is a *dignified* way to eat in company. Would you use one?

Walking-aids and wheelchairs. Sticks, tripods, walking-frames, wheeling trolleys – the list is endless, and it is essential to get specialist advice when choosing aids of this type. Make sure there is space in the user's home to manoeuvre the aid around from one room to another. It is also essential to teach the person how to use it and when to discard it when it is no longer necessary. Walking-frames are addictive, and even when the person has re-established balancing and walking skills they may carry their frame in front of them like a mascot.

Wheelchairs can be self-propelling, push-chairs or electrically operated. For a mentally frail person you must get one that is safe for them to be left sitting in without it running away at the push of a button, but light and easily manoeuvred by the person giving a helping hand.

Incontinence aids. Protective garments and liners, adaptations to clothing, male and female urinals, male appliances with tubing, bed pads, furniture protection – all are widely available, but again, get expert advice. Many aids centres have an advisory service on incontinence.

Clothing. The invention of Velcro as a substitute fastener makes wrap-over skirts and trousers much easier to take on and off. Front-opening garments, wide sleeves and stretchy neck openings all make dressing easier. There is plenty of special clothing on the market, but with common sense it is also possible to adapt ordinary clothing. Why, however, do the specialised clothing manufacturers think that disabled people want to look like frumps? What we need are *stylish*, modern clothes that are easily laundered and do not look like 'regulation issue'.

Beware: some aids not usually useful for mentally frail people. Many aids become indispensable and can make life much easier for patients and those caring for them. But there are also a number of superficially attractive aids that are *not* useful for elderly people with confusion or dementia. Beware of any gadget that the person has to *learn to use*, e.g. electric can-openers, new-style jug electric kettles, a new electric fire, central heating or a new telephone.

Practically all alarm-call systems are useless for mentally frail patients. The only ones a relative may find useful are those that do not depend on the user to activate them but respond passively to some action of the person. There is for example an alarm that you can place under a bed mat or under the carpet on the door threshold; when someone treads on it, this will sound a warning signal in another room. This can be useful to indicate when a confused person is wandering or needs to find the bathroom. The vast majority of alarms, however, depend on the wearer pressing a button or activating a switch when they need help. A confused person will either fail to activate the alarm when in need or activate it repeatedly to the irritation of the person on the receiving end of multiple false emergency calls.

9

Depression

No one these days seems to talk about feeling sad or unhappy. Events and circumstances are described as 'sad', but we usually describe people as feeling 'low', 'miserable', 'fed up' or 'depressed'. We all pass through times in our lives when nothing seems to go right. Circumstances seem somehow to 'gang up' on us; the future looks bleak. Feeling upset and low is a natural response to adversity and can sometimes have a beneficial effect by sparking off a determination to take stock of a bad situation, rethink priorities and make alternative plans for the future. This is the healthy reaction to life's problems that we call 'coming to terms with things'. Depression and unhappiness can therefore be entirely understandable sequels to unhappy events that people need time to get over.

Depression in the medical sense, however, means something very different from just feeling understandably low spirited or fed up. The more severe forms of depression are real illnesses and are characterised not only by low 'mood' but also by certain specific physical symptoms. These more serious forms of depression are referred to by psychiatrists as 'depressive illnesses' or 'depressive disorders'. Depressions of this kind cause an enormous amount of suffering to the afflicted person and their family. This chapter describes the way depression affects older people and what can be done about it.

How common is depression in elderly people?

Old age is commonly regarded as the season of sorrow and despair. One stereotyped view of old age is that depression and misery are the predictable, understandable response to the losses and declines of the last period of life. Young people especially tend to view their future old age gloomily. They expect the worst and believe misery and despair to be the natural product of old age. In fact, however, the vast majority of elderly people are not depressed or miserable at all and no more of them suffer from depressive illnesses than do younger people. It is nevertheless important to remember that a significant minority, perhaps one in ten, of the population do suffer from depression; this poses an enormous burden on families and causes the sufferers a great deal of mental anguish.

It is extremely important to spot when someone is depressed because depression is *treatable*, by a variety of means. Severe depression usually gets better when treated with the right medicines, and there is a great deal that family and friends can do to help.

Depression in people living in old people's homes and nursing homes

Old people living in old people's homes or nursing homes are more likely to suffer from depression than people living in their own homes. As many as one-third of the residents of such homes in Britain are suffering in this way. We do not know if the environment and quality of life in these institutions are the cause of the problem. Many of our old people's homes certainly have a depressing atmosphere about them; which of us would care to live in one? Alternatively it is possible that elderly people who are already depressed enter old people's homes in an attempt to solve their problems, seeking out a more supportive and sheltered environment, relieved of the worries of managing at home on their own. Entering a home is not unfortunately an effective treatment for depression and rarely solves the problem. The move may well serve to reinforce a depressed person's sense of inferiority and uselessness. The staff do not have the advantage of knowing what the elderly individual's personality was like before the depression began and sometimes assume that the person was always that way. Staff are unlikely under these circumstances to seek professional help to improve the person's outlook and often do not expect the individual to recover.

It is difficult to ignore the distress of a depressed person who is living in a family. Everyone around them feels tense, under strain and painfully aware of the problem. This is not the case in a large old people's home, however, where residents who become withdrawn and self-preoccupied may scarcely be noticed as behaving unusually. But depressed people feel *desperate* and they try to communicate this despair and need for help in some way. One way to draw attention to their plight is to behave in an awkward, rebellious way, demanding time and attention from staff by asking for more physical care and help. Incontinence, inability to walk unaided and bad-tempered or aggressive outbursts towards other residents and staff may all be symptoms of depression. Complaining, hypochondriacal and irritable elderly people are frequently suffering from depression.

Signs that a person has depression

A depressed person is not just someone who is feeling low-spirited. In fact that is one of the least likely reasons for the condition. Depression affects every part of the person's thinking, feeling, conversation, behaviour and physical health. Specific symptoms often give the clue to the diagnosis. The main clue to look for is a definite *change* over the course of days or weeks from being an active, coping and competent person to being a different sort of personality. It may take weeks or months for family and friends to appreciate the great change that has come about in their relative. It is easy to attribute the change to 'just old age'. If someone's personality appears to change for the worse, and the change persists for several weeks, then professional help should be sought.

Turning now to individual symptoms, it is worth noting first that there is an enormous variation from one depressed person to another, and the symptoms will not all be present at once.

Mood

Feelings of depression are *unpleasant*. Although sometimes there is a straightforward feeling of being sad, low and dispirited, more often the mood is one of being keyed up, tense and extremely *anxious* for no apparent reason. Depressed people feel fatigued and generally unwell. Waves of panicky fear sweep over them, and there is a foreboding of impending catastrophe without any identifiable cause. Some people feel dreadfully ill and worn out all day. *Feeling ill and anxious makes people very irritable.* They snap at other people, complain about noise and feel constantly 'on a short fuse'. The fearfulness of depression makes them cling to other people and constantly seek help and reassurance. This anxious, clinging behaviour can be extremely annoying for those around them, and most relatives and friends find it difficult to feel sympathetic towards a depressed person.

Someone with a serious depressive illness usually feels much worse first thing in the morning, but then brightens up a little as the day wears on. However, others may feel progressively more despondent and worried with every passing hour and quite worn out by the end of the day.

Depressed thoughts

Depressed people feel as though they are looking at the world from the bottom of a dark pit from which they can never escape. The future appears hopelessly gloomy; they feel they will never recover. Thoughts of death intrude in an unpleasant way, and most depressed people at some point wish they were dead: 'I wish the Lord would take me one night'; or 'I wouldn't care if a bus ran me over.' These fleeting notions of wanting life to be over are very common in all depressed people. Some go much further and actively consider means of doing away with themselves. Elderly people, especially men, are more likely to commit suicide than younger people. Even so, suicide is very rare. Most depressed elderly people are too closely attached to their friends and relatives to hurt them in this way. The knowledge of how their family and friends would feel when they found out about the suicide is one of the main reasons why depressed people struggle on with life.

Depressed people interpret everything they hear or observe in a gloomy way. They feel inferior to other people and that they are worthless, no good to anyone. Some sufferers tend to blame other people for their problems and act in a suspicious, unfriendly and hostile way. Others feel deeply ashamed and guilty for no apparent reason. They feel they have a responsibility for some 'catastrophe' due to a previous misdeed.

When an elderly person develops severe depression, they may begin to believe all manner of peculiar things. For example, they may become convinced that their home is falling apart and in a dilapidated state, that the heating and domestic appliances are broken, that they have sunk into poverty and debt, that they are responsible for a serious catastrophe in their family as a result of their wickedness. The sufferer often attributes all the symptoms to serious physical illness, which they believe is untreatable and from which they will shortly die. Cancer, venereal disease and brain tumour are perhaps the three commonest illnesses that depressed patients fear. They cannot be reassured that all is well no matter how much time is spent trying to persuade them. Similarly, no amount of 'proof' will persuade a depressed person that their ideas are false once the ideas have become firmly rooted. Depressed people are so preoccupied with their own gloomy thoughts that they find it hard to take an interest in things going on around them.

This makes them appear lazy and selfish to other people. They lose interest in their family, friends and home and yet at the same time desperately want someone to be with them.

Activity

Depression brings tiredness, fatigue and a feeling of being lethargic and lacking in energy. This 'slowing down' makes people withdrawn and uncommunicative. They speak more slowly than usual and in short, uninformative sentences. A depressed person may be so 'slowed up' that they appear to lack understanding. It is almost as if they were suffering from dementia. On the other hand, depressed people can be extremely restless and agitated. Depressed elderly people sometimes find it impossible to sit still for any length of time and feel unable to concentrate on anything – their mind jumps from one worry to the next. Losing the ability to concentrate makes sufferers feel as if they are losing their memories, and they often wonder if they are losing their minds and becoming demented. No wonder that it is sometimes difficult for both relatives and professionals to tell the difference between depression and dementia.

There *is* a difference, however. With depression, housework gets neglected, no task is ever finished, and day-to-day life seems impossibly difficult. There is a never-ending and unsuccessful struggle to get things done. Nevertheless there is an essential underlying capability to do things. With dementia, on the other hand, this ability is eroded. Fragments, even large fragments, of ability remain, but the overall capacity to get things done no longer exists.

Sleep

Elderly people often sleep less at night than younger people. They tend to catch up during the day through cat-napping for short periods. Elderly people today also tend to belong to a generation that traditionally started work early in the morning, so it is not unusual for the habit of rising at six o'clock or earlier to persist long into retirement. However, depressed people have great difficulty getting off to sleep; they tend to wake frequently through the night and then wake early in the morning feeling unrefreshed and still tired. Waking regularly at three or four in the morning feeling frightened and despairing is a particular sign of serious depression.

Appetite

Some people with mild depression keep eating the same as usual although they may have lost enjoyment in their meals. But most depressed people lose their appetite. It is not just that they do not feel like eating, but taking food itself becomes unpleasant, and it becomes difficult to get it down. Food seems to stick in the throat or give an unpleasant over-full feeling. Consequently one of the key signs of depression is *weight loss*. This can sometimes be very dramatic, and a loss of a stone or more over the course of a few weeks is not uncommon. (Serious weight loss can also be due to physical illness: see Chapter 8.)

Bowels

Constipation is almost universal in depression. An overall slowing down and loss of appetite lead to a slowing of the bowels too. Some people become so preoccupied with their bowel function that they can think and talk of nothing else, an irritating symptom for those who have to listen to 'blow-by-blow' accounts of bowel actions every day.

Other physical symptoms

Increased tension in the body muscles leads to numerous aches and pains. Severe headaches, which feel like a tight band round the head or a weight on top of the head, neck-aches and backaches are all common. Anxiety leads to episodes of dizziness, giddiness, churning stomach, cold sweats and breathlessness. These symptoms can be very hard to distinguish from real physical disease, and it is not surprising that sufferers frequently interpret them as being caused by physical illness.

Two brief descriptions will give an idea of the different kinds of depression common in old age:

Annie Brown. Widowed ten years ago, she lives alone on the third floor of a block of flats in a Glasgow suburb. Over the last five years she has become less mobile because of arthritis in her knees and now walks only with the aid of a frame. She never goes out alone because she can't get upstairs and downstairs by herself, and the flats have no lift. She is in considerable pain most of the time. The pills her doctor prescribed for her arthritis give her indigestion, so she doesn't take them regularly. The doctor told her that her knees would improve if she lost weight, but food is one of the few pleasures left to her. She sees her home help twice a week for an hour and relies on her to do all the shopping and housework. They don't always see eye to eye, however, because Mrs Brown is irritable, grumbles at the price of food and blames her help for not finding better bargains. The home help finds Mrs Brown one of her less sympathetic clients and is relieved to be off at the end of the hour. She is fed up with her client's constant grumbling and seemingly continuous preoccupation with her own aches and pains. For Mrs Brown the days seem endlessly long; she sleeps poorly and spends long hours mulling over the past when she and her husband enjoyed life together. She hopes that she will die soon, just not wake up one morning. She has never told anyone how low she feels, and no one has ever asked.

Fred Smith. Two years ago, at the age of sixty-eight, he had a stroke. He made a good physical recovery and, although he sometimes drags his right leg after walking a long way, most people wouldn't notice there was anything wrong. However, his wife has noticed a change in him over the past two years. He is generally slower, cries at the least little thing and is embarrassingly tearful in public if he meets an old friend or relative. His wife is puzzled by this but accepts it as a result of the stroke. Two months ago there

was a rapid deterioration in Mr Smith's mood. He has
become withdrawn and morose, sits for long hours staring
into space doing nothing, has lost interest in the snooker on
TV and hardly speaks when spoken to. He eats very little
and has lost nearly a stone in weight. At night he sleeps
very poorly and wakes early in the small hours. He
occasionally mutters about the terrible poverty he feels they
have fallen into and repeatedly asks to look at the bank
statement and pension book. Mrs Smith cannot reassure
him that all is well. He ruminates about the dilapidated state
of the house and about the garden becoming overgrown. In
the early hours of the morning he plots how he might kill
himself and wonders what terrible fate would befall his wife
if he were to leave her alone.

Mr Smith and Mrs Brown have different kinds of
depression. It is much easier to understand how lonely,
isolated Mrs Brown could have become depressed, but more
difficult to spot that the problem is depression. It is not at all
straightforward to understand Mr Smith's depression,
which seems to have come out of the blue and has now
become a very serious condition. However, most people
would recognise that Mr Smith is depressed and ill and
needs treatment.

Telling the difference between depression and dementia

Dementia sufferers are not normally very concerned about
their failing mental powers and rarely complain of memory
loss. Depressed people on the other hand often complain of
memory difficulties. The memory problems of depression
are due to loss of concentration – so that the person cannot
take in what is said to them – not to loss of memory
function.

Also, depression is a painful, distressing condition for the
sufferer, whereas dementia normally causes more suffering
to immediate relatives than to the person affected.
Depressed people are gloomy, sad and withdrawn, and can

think only of unhappy things. Demented people do not concentrate on any one thing at all; although their mood may be changeable, they are not usually continuously unhappy. Serious loss of appetite and complaints of insomnia are commoner with depression than with dementia.

A further point: *it is possible to suffer from both dementia and depression at the same time*. Dementia often appears worse than it really is because of depression. It is important to spot depression in a dementia sufferer because treating the depression can make a marked difference to the person's ability to think clearly and optimistically and make best use of their failing mental abilities.

What causes depression in the elderly?

The answer to this is not as simple as it may seem. When people feel low they can normally identify the cause relatively easily. A bereavement, a close friend moving away or serious ill health affecting someone we love are obvious reasons for feeling distressed and upset. The quality all these circumstances share is that they are losses, or threatened losses. The elderly are more at risk than younger people of being bereaved of close friends and relatives but they are also more likely to suffer from other important losses. Loss of physical health, loss of mobility making it difficult to get out of the house, and loss of one's own home on entering residential care are common examples. Some depressed elderly people have experienced a serious bereavement in the recent past. It may however have occurred several months earlier and may not be recognised as the cause by the person concerned. Moreover, a person who has been depressed for months or years may have long forgotten the factor that triggered off the problem in the first place.

In part our personalities determine whether we react badly or not to adverse circumstances. Some people suffer from 'nerves' all their lives. They are inclined to over-react with excessive worry to the least problem. 'Worriers' and 'highly strung' people are more likely to get depressed than lifelong optimists.

One of the most important causes of depression is long-standing poor physical health. Chronic pain, immobility and feeling 'under the weather' are understandable causes of depression. Someone who is taking a lot of tablets for heart and chest problems or arthritis often feels permanently 'off colour'. Serious depression can nevertheless come quite suddenly, with no apparent cause at all. We do not know why some people are liable to develop depression of this kind, but it is possible that changes in the biochemistry of the ageing brain predispose some individuals to developing depression.

What can be done?

The most important thing that a friend or relative can do for a depressed person is to *spot* that the person has become depressed and ask the family doctor to assess whether or not they need medical treatment with antidepressant medication or other physical treatments.

Medical treatment for depression

The notion that depression can be helped by medication may seem strange. After all, if the cause was a long-standing spell in hospital with a painful illness, you might expect that once the cause was removed the person would recover their good spirits. You might also expect that people would come to terms eventually with bereavement and other serious losses. Most people do recover from this kind of demoralisation or grief without medical intervention, but sometimes the depression takes on a life of its own and persists beyond what others feel to be a reasonable time. In a sense the patient gets 'set' and cannot return to normal, even when the cause of the depression is long gone.

Depressive illness is associated with an upset in the

brain's metabolism. Medication can reverse this upset and return the person to normal. Medication cannot reverse normal unhappiness, of course, or control the normal grief of bereavement, but it can help in those cases of serious depression where appetite and sleep are affected or where the person has become very agitated or slowed down.

Tranquilliser drugs such as diazepam (Valium) or lorazepam (Ativan) are *not* antidepressants. They merely act as temporary sedatives and mask the underlying problem. They should never be prescribed to a depressed person unless the doctor has decided to use them in conjunction with one of the true antidepressants.

Antidepressant drugs take at least ten days and sometimes as long as three to four weeks before they begin to work. It can be very tedious taking tablets regularly every day when no benefit is detected. Plenty of perseverence is required of the patient. Relatives can help considerably by encouraging the person regularly. A small dose is usually prescribed first and then the dose is built up over the course of a week. Like all medication, antidepressant drugs may have unpleasant, unwanted effects that can be troublesome and need watching out for. But it is worth persevering because they really can help enormously.

Antidepressant drugs are *not addictive* and can be stopped after the end of the course of treatment without unwanted effects. A course of antidepressant drugs lasts from six months to two or three years, and is usually continued after the symptoms of depression have lifted. This is because depression in elderly people tends to recur within a few months if the medication is withdrawn early.

Side-effects of antidepressant drugs. The list of unwanted effects is long. Most people experience the less serious ones very mildly, but it is as well to be aware of them.

(1) Dizziness, especially when rising from a chair or getting out of bed.
(2) Difficulty in starting the stream when passing urine.
(3) Dry mouth.

(4) Constipation.
(5) Difficulty in focusing the eyes.
(6) Sleepiness: this can be put to good effect by taking most of the tablets at night.
(7) Mental confusion: this occurs in some vulnerable elderly people and is an indication that the medication should be stopped immediately and a doctor consulted. He may wish to restart the drug at a lower dose.

Most antidepressant medicines are dangerous if taken in overdose. There is a danger that a depressed person will take them as a means of suicide. If someone has expressed suicidal ideas, however fleeting or seemingly unimportant, they should never be left to supervise their own medication. A relative or friend should keep the bottle of tablets and give only one or two days' supply at a time. The person should be told why this is being done and will often be relieved of the burden of having an easy means of self-poisoning in the house.

How else can relatives and friends help?

One important fact is worth remembering: *nearly all depressed people get better in time*. Treatment speeds up the process, but nature will eventually heal the problem. During the period of depression, relatives can help enormously by continually reminding the person that they will feel better in time and of the good and successful things in their lives. Relatives and friends should also remember to tell the sufferer that someone cares about them.

It is easy to fall into a pattern of behaviour with a depressed person that is rejecting and unhelpful. When someone is irritable, rude and complaining towards you when you visit, for example, it is tempting to visit less frequently in future and to ignore the person, hoping they will appreciate you more following an absence. But this will make a depressed person feel even more rejected and isolated. Try to avoid telling someone who feels very ill that 'there's nothing the matter with you' when they persistently complain about headaches or other bodily ailments. On the other hand, it will not be helpful to pursue endless complaints in enormous detail and plague the doctor or nurse with yet more symptoms that are part of the depression and not due to physical illness. Try to steer a middle course and avoid extremes of attitude. Do not pretend to go along with delusional ideas, but do not argue either or try to prove the ideas false. Colluding with false beliefs is acting dishonestly while on the other hand arguing with a deluded person has no effect at all – except to make you upset.

Dissuade a depressed person from making major decisions during the course of the illness. This is not the time to decide to enter an old people's home, change a will, sell the house or move in permanently with a relative. The individual concerned often later regrets decisions made in haste while feeling depressed.

During the course of a depression it is difficult to tackle any underlying problems of isolation and loneliness because the illness itself prevents the sufferer from being able to benefit from increased social contact by forming new acquaintances and friendships. However, when someone is beginning to recover they may be more receptive to the idea of joining a club or attending a day centre to expand their social horizons. This possibility can be investigated by contacting the local area social services office.

Elderly people often lose their family contacts and friendships during the course of a depression because people lack understanding as to why the depressed person is behaving in such a difficult way. Supporting someone through a depression is a taxing and difficult business but very rewarding when the depression finally lifts and the person returns to their former self.

Bereavement

Elderly people are much more likely to be bereaved of those closest to them than younger people. As more people live out their full life span of three score years and ten or more, many people never experience the grief of losing a parent or close relative until they are in late middle age. We no longer expect young people to experience grief, and most of our society has become unfamiliar with how the bereaved person feels and how best to help them during the difficult period after the loss.

There is some suggestion from a number of studies that older people cope on the whole just as well as younger subjects when a husband or wife dies, especially when the death has been anticipated by a lengthy illness. Nevertheless some losses are especially stressful in old age, particularly the death of a grown-up son or daughter. The bereaved person often feels cruelly cheated, and life can come to seem completely meaningless.

Grief is a very stressful experience. It is usual for the sufferer to feel physically unwell for many months. There are phases of grief, and most people go through them at their own pace. Some people take only weeks to feel physically better, but the majority need several months; and it is not unusual for symptoms of grief to continue for two years or more.

Numbness

When the news first breaks, a sense of unreality and a numb lack of feeling are aroused that last for minutes, hours or a few days. The news sometimes does not seem to be taken in; the person finds it hard to believe that anything untoward has happened. While in this dazed, numbed condition the bereaved person is likely to need help with the simplest decisions. The individual also needs time – time to sit back and organise her ideas and take in what has happened. The first task of relatives and friends therefore is to help with what must be done. This includes the notification of other relatives, organising the funeral and registration of the death. The more contact with friends and relatives at this stage the better. They are often keen to give practical help, and it is a great deal easier for close friends and relatives to express their sympathy and understanding during the early days than weeks or months later.

Bereaved people in this numb phase feel lost and helpless. They often need someone to take charge of organising the routine of daily life.

Acute grief

This is a *physical* problem. The person feels tense, stressed, panicky, restless and fearful. They are highly strung and on edge. They are also physiologically over-aroused; their heart beats too fast, and muscle tension causes aches, pains and tension headaches. Sweatiness, loss of appetite and sleeplessness are also common, as is a dry mouth, indigestion, a lump in the throat and a feeling of 'food sticking in the gullet'. The person feels jumpy, bad tempered, irritable and easily upset. At the same time as suffering these physically upsetting feelings, waves of acute longing for the dead person occur. These 'pangs' of grief come over the person in waves, often out of the blue, several times a day. Such tensions and feelings of ill health can last for many months and it is not uncommon for them to persist in elderly people up to two years after losing a husband or wife.

Persistent and obtrusive pangs of yearning and pining for the person who is gone represent a kind of searching for that loved person. Some people find crying very difficult at this stage; tears seem bottled up inside and will not come out. As by this time the person feels preoccupied with thoughts of the dead loved one to the exclusion of everything else, this makes concentrating on other things very difficult indeed. Housework and keeping up a good personal appearance are often carried out in a mechanical, meaningless way from habit and from a sense of duty.

Bereaved people often gain comfort from a feeling or impression that the dead person is near by. This comforting 'sense of presence', of spiritual nearness, is so strong for some people that they are sure they hear the dead person's voice or mistakenly feel they have 'seen' the person. These illusions are usually welcome and comforting, and relatives should not worry about such odd experiences or dissuade the person if the experiences seem very real. The illusions gradually recede over a period of weeks or months.

As the months go by

Gradually the pain diminishes, and the pangs become less frequent. Recollections of good times flood the person in a nostalgic, bitter-sweet way. Dreams become a little happier. Strangely it is at this time that feelings of irritability and anger may set in. The first overwhelmingly angry feeling is of protest and bitterness against those who allowed the death to happen – the hospital doctor who was thoughtless, the GP who didn't come quickly enough, the sister-in-law who should have visited that day, and so on. Anger is closely allied to a sense of guilt that the bereaved person did not do enough or would have averted the tragedy 'if only . . .'

What can relatives do to help?

After the funeral is over the people who are most valued are those who stick around to help in a practical way and accept without reproach the tendency of the bereaved person to pour out feelings of anguish and sometimes anger, even if this is directed against the helper. The bereaved person should feel that they do not have to 'bottle up' their distress, or on the other hand talk excessively about it, if they do not want to. Over-insistent 'probing' may be just as bad as 'jollying' along or trying to avoid upsetting the person. Grief cannot be evaded. Relatives can help by pointing out that these overwhelming feelings are normal and not a sign of madness or illness.

It is often a few weeks after the funeral that difficulties arise in the family. Children often feel they want to shelter an elderly bereaved parent, for example by helping them move house. This is the time when elderly people are most likely to move in with their children or make a hasty decision to move to a home. But this is a time for children to *watch and wait* and allow the elderly person to make up his or her own mind. Realising the loss fully, accepting it and planning a new life can take from one to three years or even more. Curiously, the closer and better the relationship between two people, the better and more complete the eventual adjustment often is. This is because when two people love each other deeply, one partner becomes 'incorporated' into the other person's mind as a living memory. Widows of such relationships often eventually feel that 'I cannot ever lose him now; he has become a part of me.'

An elderly bereaved parent often has to renegotiate relationships with the adult children. The widow may feel the children owe her more attention and time now than when both parents were alive. This can cause resentment on the part of the children at the extra demand on their affections. In such circumstances the bereaved individual is often someone with no close 'affectional' ties to friends, neighbours or other relatives. She therefore tends to focus on her children for all emotional support. Children cannot do a great deal about this extra demand except help the person to make social links outside the immediate family circle and be firm but fair about providing extra help at this difficult time.

Mourning takes time. The key to understanding and helping a bereaved elderly person is to allow time to heal the grief. This means weeks, months or sometimes years. Mourning cannot be rushed, especially in old age.

Can anyone else help?

In some areas, *bereavement counselling schemes* are run by voluntary organisations such as Age Concern or by local social work departments. These schemes are badly named, since most people do not want 'counselling' – which smacks of patronising do-gooders telling bereaved people what is good for them. What such schemes are really about is simply a befriending process for bereaved people who *want* to talk about their loss and their troubles to a sympathetic person who knows something of the common problems that a bereaved person faces. Many people do find them useful; sometimes it is much easier to confide in a friendly stranger than in a member of the family who may be having their own difficulties adjusting to the loss. On the other hand, those who find talking over problems difficult at any time are unlikely to reap any benefit from them, so never push someone into going to a scheme such as this if they are reluctant.

10

Paranoid Conditions

'Paranoid' means 'believing in wrong ideas' or being deluded. The term has often been used colloquially to describe people who are over-sensitive and suspicious, because often the incorrect beliefs that people hold are of being persecuted or harmed by others. Paranoid conditions are relatively rare in elderly people; only about one in a hundred elderly people suffers from them. Such mental disorders are sometimes referred to as *paraphrenia* and are sometimes regarded as a late-onset form of schizophrenia, the serious mental disorder that usually affects younger people.

Symptoms of paranoid illness

The main symptom is a fixed delusion that the individual is being threatened, harassed, abused or persecuted in some way. This delusion is not susceptible to reason or argument. The commonest forms of this delusion are that the neighbours are trying to take over the house, that people are plotting to steal money and possessions or that the individual is being sexually molested. The beliefs are nearly always bizarre and quite unbelievable to anyone thinking in a rational way. One patient I knew believed that a neighbour was beaming X-rays through the walls, causing the furniture to be rearranged and damaged. Another patient insisted that a woman who lived down the road had a gang of policemen under her control who came into the patient's house at night and sexually molested her. Yet another believed that she could smell gas coming up through the floorboards that was ruining her health.

The delusional belief is sometimes triggered in the sufferer's mind by the mind's attempt to 'explain' another distressing symptom, that of hearing noises and voices. The noise that sufferers hear is often a 'shushing' or 'engine-like' noise but can be bells, music, recognisable songs or hymns, sounding very loud to the person. These strange noises often seem to be based on *tinnitus*, a distressing ringing noise that is produced in an ageing ear. Patients often describe it as a 'ringing in the ears' or as 'grating noises'. It is quite easy to understand how these noises could be distorted so as to become recognisable sounds or voices. Such voices may sometimes be heard talking to the individual in an abusive way, referring to her as a 'whore' or as evil. The paranoid individual occasionally hears several 'voices' having a conversation about her or commenting on her actions – 'She's having a cup of tea now. Now she's going out shopping. She's getting the milk off the doorstep', and so on – often in an accusatory or disparaging fashion.

These extraordinary phenomena are very distressing for the sufferer, to whom they are frighteningly real and threatening. The individual is *mentally alert* and is *not suffering from dementia*. She is usually able to care for herself just as well as before the onset of the illness.

The individual's attempts to deal with this frightening situation often draw other people's attention to her plight. The local police, the gas board, the electricity board or the neighbours may be bombarded with complaints or verbal and physical abuse. One patient of mine, persistently distressed by loud music from what she believed to be her neighbours' 'juke-boxes' that 'played all night', got up at three o'clock one morning and angrily hurled half a dozen empty milk bottles through both sets of neighbours' bedroom windows, to the astonishment of the sleeping couples next door.

Who develops a paranoid illness?

The victim of this distressing illness is usually a woman who has lived alone for many years, frequently a single person or a long-widowed, fairly isolated person. She is often someone who has preferred her own company and made few friends. The illness occasionally develops in someone who has always been a bit suspicious, inclined to take against people easily or be readily offended, but this is not a universal rule. There are many sufferers who have been friendly, trusting people and who develop the symptoms seemingly for no reason.

Severe deafness, usually present for twenty years or more, afflicts about half of the sufferers of this type of paranoia. Tinnitus often goes along with the deafness. Poor sight is another common accompaniment, sometimes associated with visual hallucinations – seeing things that are not really there.

What can be done?

Never try to argue or reason with someone with delusions. You will become just one more person who does not believe the story and makes them feel even more isolated and friendless. On the other hand, you must try to avoid giving the impression that you can hear the noise, see the vision or truly believe that she is being persecuted. The most helpful response is to imply that you sympathise and understand the problem, that you are on her side and will do everything to help her out of this predicament. *The single most important thing you can do to help is persuade her to see her doctor*, because the illness can be helped, and sometimes cured completely, with the right medication. It is no easy task to persuade someone who feels embattled and defensive to see a doctor. Never imply that you think she is mentally disordered or tell her that she is 'imagining things'. Try instead to explain that you are worried about the effect her 'troubles' are having on her general health and that you would like her to have a check-up. Needless to say, you had better warn the doctor first what the real problem is. A physical check-up is a good idea in any case, because on rare occasions paranoid states develop secondary to a physical illness such as an under-active thyroid gland.

Be sure to make contact with the neighbours or who-ever is bearing the brunt of your relative's wrong beliefs. They often have to put up with their walls or doors being bashed at all hours or with being abused over the garden fence. One of my patients, believing that her prized roses had been poisoned by the neighbours, went round one afternoon and cut the heads off all her neighbour's roses. Enlisting the tolerance and support of the other 'victims' of the illness is important; people are often surprisingly understanding if the real causes of the problems are explained.

Hearing and sight

If possible, persuade the person to have her hearing and sight tested. Do it tactfully so as not to imply that 'hearing things' is due to faulty hearing or that visions are due to faulty sight. Paranoid people do not believe it.

Medication

The most effective tablets for the treatment of paranoid illnesses are thioridazine (Melleril), chlorpromazine (Largactil) and trifluoperazine (Stelazine). Taken regularly in the right dosage, these drugs usually cause the symptoms to disappear in a week or two. However, there are problems with such medicines. First, patients often do not want to take them and become suspicious; so 'non-compliance' – refusing to take them in the right dose – is a common problem. Moreover, the drugs can give very unpleasant side-effects. Elderly women develop these more frequently than elderly men or younger people. Unwanted effects are tremor, stiffness, slurred speech, an unpleasant urge to move around, drowsiness, a tendency to fall, dry mouth and constipation. If taken for a long time these medicines can cause unpleasant rhythmic movements of the facial muscles and limbs. Not everyone suffers these side-effects, and it is usually possible to adjust the dose so as to minimise the unwanted effects yet at the same time give maximum benefit to the patient. There are also tablets that counteract the unwanted effects, which can be taken in conjunction with the active tablets.

Because of the reluctance of many patients to take tablets or medicine regularly, injectable medicines have been developed that need only to be given once every month. The commonest of these injectable drugs are fluphenazine (Modecate) and flupenthixol (Depixol). The GP may give the injection himself or he may ask a community psychiatric nurse to call regularly to give the injection at home.

A CPN (community psychiatric nurse) can be valuable in the management of an elderly person with a paranoid illness. Over a period of regular visits a nurse can often persuade the sufferer to accept medication by injection and can also tackle the other relevant problems, such as isolation and loneliness.

Measures to tackle isolation

People with paranoid illnesses often spend long hours alone in their own homes behind locked and bolted doors. It is sometimes impossible to persuade them to give up their self-imposed isolation, and all one can do is to keep visiting regularly, always maintaining a friendly tone of voice – although the only response may be through the letter-box! Some people, however, are able to recognise their own loneliness and crave the company of others. They may be willing to be introduced to a day centre, a luncheon club or drop-in centre. It is in this area that relatives working with a community psychiatric nurse can often achieve a lot to relieve the conditions that may have predisposed to the development of the illness.

'She wants to move. What shall we do?'

The deluded sufferer very often wishes to solve her problem by moving away from the neighbourhood where she feels persecuted. It is frequently only after several moves from one house to another that relatives or the housing authority recognise that the constant urge to get away from unfriendly neighbours is a symptom of a paranoid illness. Moving house does not generally solve the problem at all. The patient merely transfers her delusional ideas to her new neighbours or mysteriously discovers that the old persecutors have found ways of influencing her over a great distance by means of X-rays or electricity wires.

'Can't we insist she has treatment?'

Persuading a person with a paranoid illness to accept treatment, particularly medication, can be a tiring and fruitless business. In Britain you cannot insist that a patient accepts treatment against her own wishes unless the patient's physical health is seriously at risk or she is putting others at risk of harm. Under these circumstances the patient may be admitted to a hospital under a compulsory order for treatment. The details of the Mental Health Act orders, how they are used and under what circumstances are discussed in Chapter 7. Most doctors and social workers are extremely reluctant to admit an elderly patient on a compulsory order and use this route to help the patient only when other ways have failed and when a crisis makes an admission imperative to protect the patient's health. *Causing a public nuisance is not sufficient justification for a compulsory admission.* Neighbours can of course bring a civil action against the person if their lives are seriously upset by noise or if there is damage to their property.

Points to ponder

When the elderly person is distressed, frightened or saddened by her delusional ideas it is surely right to offer help with medication and all the supports one can offer. Furthermore, where neighbours' lives are being made miserable by her accusations it is worth trying to intervene to help. But quite often the patient remains quite cheerful, copes well, is not really bothered by her bizarre beliefs and doesn't interfere with anyone else. Under these circumstances it may be kinder to leave the illness untreated because of the difficulties in getting the medication right.

Paranoid individuals do not usually want to enter residential care. They are independent people unused to the company of others and often do not react well to living in a group. Even when you are concerned for a paranoid loved one's health it is generally better to try to tackle the problem in her home than to remove her permanently into an old people's home.

Appendix: Useful Organisations, Their Addresses and What They Do

Organisations listed here will provide information, advice and in some cases practical support to elderly people and their families. Most are charities that depend on donations to finance their work, so they normally make a small charge for membership and for larger leaflets. They nevertheless offer an enormous amount of free advice too, so do write to them if you feel they may have something to offer you. Many have local branches – look them up in your local telephone directory.

Age Concern England   Tel. 01-640 5431
Information Department
60 Pitcairn Road
Mitcham, Surrey
CR4 3LL

Useful leaflets and publications on a host of subjects. Many local branches doing valuable work with mentally frail elderly people.

Alzheimer's Disease Society   Tel. 01-381 3177
Bank Buildings
Fulham Broadway
London SW6 1EP

The organisation for all sufferers and relatives of *any kind* of dementia, whatever the age of the sufferer. Growing fast, many local branches and self-help support groups for relatives. Also has a medical research fund if *you* want to give a donation. Useful booklets providing information and advice.

Arthritis Care   Tel. 01-235 0902
6 Grosvenor Crescent
London SW1X 7ER

A charity concerned with the welfare of arthritis sufferers.

Association of Carers   Tel. 0634-813981/2
58 New Road
Chatham, Kent
ME4 4QR

An advice service plus newsletters and local self-help groups for anyone caring for a dependent person.

Association of Crossroads Care   Tel. 0788-73653
Attendant Schemes Ltd
94 Coton Road
Rugby, Warwickshire
CV21 4LN

Growing number of local groups providing practical help for the carers of physically handicapped people of all ages. Some groups are able to offer a service to physically and mentally frail elderly people.

British Diabetic Association   Tel. 01-323 1531
10 Queen Anne Street
London W1M 0BD

Advice and information on diabetes.

British Heart Foundation   Tel. 01-935 0185
102 Gloucester Place
London W1H 4DH

Pamphlets on heart problems and stroke.

British Talking Book Service for the Blind   Tel. 01-903 6666
Mount Pleasant
Wembley, Middlesex
HAQ 1RR

Loans of machines and tapes for an annual subscription.

Chest, Heart and Stroke Association   Tel. 01-387 3012
Tavistock House North
Tavistock Square
London WC1H 9JE

Also has branches in Scotland and Northern Ireland. Useful information on strokes, heart disease, chest complaints of all kinds including bronchitis, emphysema and asthma.

Counsel and Care for the Elderly   Tel. 01-621 1624
131 Middlesex Street
London E1 7JF

Gives information and advice for elderly people in private residential homes. Also gives grants for short stays in residential care.

Court of Protection   Tel. 01-636 6877
Chief Clerk
25 Store Street
London WC1E 7BP

Cruse   Tel. 01-940 4818/9047
Cruse House
126 Sheen Road
Richmond, Surrey
TW9 1UR

An organisation for the welfare of widowed people and their children.

Dial UK Ltd   Tel. 0246-864498
NADIAS
Victoria Buildings
117 High Street
Clay Cross, Derbyshire
S45 9DZ

Information on where to see and buy aids for living.

Disabled Living Foundation   Tel. 01-289 6111
380–384 Harrow Road
London W9 1HU

Everything you could possibly want to know about aids and where to get them. Professional advice services, especially on incontinence, clothing, mobility aids, etc.

Disablement Income Group   Tel. 01-247 2128/6877
Attlee House
28 Commercial Street
London E1 6LR

Advice on benefits and how to claim them for disabled people.

Friends of the Elderly and Gentlefolks Help   Tel. 01-730 8263
42 Ebury Street
London SW1W 0L2

Grants for repairs, heating, equipment, home nursing fees. Applications usually via a social worker.

Help the Aged   Tel. 01-253 0253
St James's Walk
London EC1R 0BE

A fund-raising charity that gives grants to other charities and organisations for projects with elderly people. Supports projects at home and abroad.

MIND (National Association for Mental Health) Tel. 01-637 0741
22 Harley Street
London W1N 2ED

A pressure group with many local branches for all sufferers
of mental disorder, whatever their age. Useful booklets and
information.

National Council for Carers and their   Tel. 01-262 1451/2
Dependants
29 Chilworth Mews
London W2 3RG

More information and advice. Many local branches.

Parkinson's Disease Society   Tel. 01-323 1174
36 Portland Place
London W1N 3DG

Information, advice, helpful leaflets. Local branches hold
regular meetings, outings, activities.

Pensioners' Voice (National Federation of
Old Age Pensioners' Associations)
Melling House
91 Preston New Road
Blackburn, Lancashire
BB2 6BD

Campaigns for welfare rights and pensions for elderly
people.

Registered Nursing Homes' Association   Tel. 01-346 1224
7a Station Road
Finchley
London N3 2SB

Publishes a list of private nursing homes belonging to the
association that have been registered by the local health
authority. This does not guarantee quality, but many of the
better nursing homes are members of the association.

Royal National Institute for the Blind   Tel. 01-388 1266
224 Great Portland Street
London W1N 6AA

Information on all eye problems, plus aids for the blind and
partially sighted.

Royal National Institute for the Deaf   Tel. 01-387 8033
105 Gower Street
London WC1E 6AH

Information and advice on hearing problems; gives grants to
other voluntary organisations.

Talking Newspapers UK   Tel. 04352-6102
68a High Street
Heathfield, East Sussex
TN21 8JB

The best of the newspapers and women's magazines on tape
several times a year.

Index